CRITICAL REALISM FOR HEALTH AND ILLNESS RESEARCH

A Practical Introduction

Priscilla Alderson

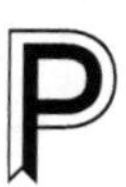

First published in Great Britain in 2021 by

Policy Press, an imprint of
Bristol University Press
University of Bristol
1-9 Old Park Hill
Bristol
BS2 8BB
UK
t: +44 (0)117 954 5940
e: bup-info@bristol.ac.uk

Details of international sales and distribution partners are available at
policy.bristoluniversitypress.co.uk

British Library Cataloguing in Publication Data
A catalogue record for this book is available from the British Library

ISBN 978-1-4473-5455-0 hardcover
ISBN 978-1-4473-5456-7 paperback
ISBN 978-1-4473-5459-8 ePub
ISBN 978-1-4473-5458-1 ePdf

Cover design: Clifford Hayes
Front cover image: Clifford Hayes

Bristol University Press and Policy Press use environmentally responsible print partners.

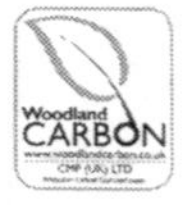

Printed in Great Britain by CMP, Poole

Contents

List of figures and tables iv
List of examples v
Acknowledgements vi

Introduction 1

1 Rethinking theories: the basis of practical research and problems with paradigms 11

2 Basic critical realist concepts 41

3 Structure and agency: making connections 65

4 Health and illness research: value-free or value-laden? 95

5 Four planes of social being: more connections 127

6 Researching transformative change over time 145

7 The point is to change it: connecting research to policy and practice 167

ABCD – Articles, books, commentary and dictionary-glossary 181

Notes 187
References 207
Index of subjects 237
Index of names 243

List of figures and tables

Figures

2.1 The semiotic triangle 44
3.1 Transformational model of social activity 85

Tables

2.1 Reducing ontology into epistemology 43
2.2 Natural necessity in physics 49
2.3 Natural necessity or the three levels of reality in life science: endocrinology 50
2.4 Natural necessity or the three levels of reality in social science: diabetes 51
2.5 Natural necessity: real, actual and empirical 51
2.6 Natural necessity and voluntary consent 60
2.7 Themes in the three dominant traditions in sociology 63
3.1 Agency, structure and natural necessity 85
4.1 Natural necessity: rights, dignity, trust and truth 109
4.2 CR levels of reality and ethics 115
4.3 Research paradigms and views of ethics 118
5.1 Laminated system for psychological research into distress 133
5.2 Barriers to interdisciplinarity and connections 138
5.3 Resolving splits between often assumed tacit theories 139
6.1 From dichotomy to dialectic 152
6.2 Feeding babies in NICU: differing perspectives 162

List of examples

1.1	Combining paradigms: an evaluation of a community-based integrated care service *Hannah Kendrick*	36
2.1	Three levels of reality in neonatal units *Rosa Mendizabal-Espinosa*	53
3.1	Using the morphogenetic cycle to evaluate a complex intervention for prison leavers with common mental health problems *Sarah Rybczynska-Bunt, Lauren Weston and Richard Byng*	86
3.2	Exploring nurses' documentation of their contribution to traumatic brain injury rehabilitation *Angela Davenport*	91
4.1	Combining critical realism with Habermas's theories *Graham Scambler*	120
5.1	Improving the physical health of people with a diagnosis of serious mental illness *Stuart Green Hofer*	130
5.2	Research into feminist-informed counselling after sexual assault *Bree Weizenegger*	132
6.1	MELD and improving care for children with allergies *Sophie Spitters*	163
7.1	Contested understandings of mental distress in the context of neoliberal reform of community mental health services in England *Rich Moth*	176

Acknowledgements

This book is based on the critical realism reading group course at the Institute of Education, University College London. The course was founded and taught by Professor Roy Bhaskar during the period 2007–14 with his friends. After Roy's death, a great loss, I became the course convenor in 2014.

I am very grateful to everyone who has shared in learning and teaching on the course and testing ideas in this book. Many of the discussions among researchers and students, on how they have applied critical realism to their work, have informed this book. Thank you to the 11 researchers who have given detailed examples of their critical realist studies.

I am also grateful to everyone who has helped me since 1972 with my research about health and illness: participants, colleagues, funders and authors in the great range of related disciplines

And thank you Alan Taman and an anonymous reviewer for very kindly commenting on the draft text and also Laura Vickers-Rendall, Amelia Watts-Jones and Millie Prekop at Policy Press, Elizabeth Stone, and the copyeditor Niranjana M N and indexer Beverley Winkler.

Introduction

> During 2020, governments faced questions about how they should work to reduce the spread of COVID-19. How should they first impose the lockdown and later manage its gradual ending? How could they protect public health while planning the slow return to 'normal' life? How could they best guide the public to cope with differences between pre- and post-pandemic views of what is 'normal' and healthy?
>
> The UK government's Scientific Advisory Group for Emergencies, SAGE, consisted mainly of scientific advisers to government departments, virologists, epidemiologists, statisticians and medical experts with risk management and 'nudge' behavioural scientists. Their expert advice varied,[1] and was widely criticised. Just as COVID-19 starkly revealed many problems in our present unequal society, it has highlighted limitations in scientific expertise and its relations to policymaking.
>
> Among innumerable policy decisions, just one example was prisons. There had long been campaigns to close many prisons. England and Wales had the largest prison population in Western Europe in April 2020, when there were plans for the early release of up to 4,000 of the 82,500 prisoners. Prison governors advised that thousands more prisoners should be released early. The aims were to reduce prison overcrowding and thereby reduce COVID-19 infection rates and deaths among prisoners and staff as well as in the communities around the prisons.
>
> Instead, only 33 prisoners were released, and in a double confinement the rest were locked up in their cells for over 23 hours a day. A prison ship and 500 shipping containers were ordered to provide extra cells. The policy increased physical and mental illness and suicide rates among already severely disadvantaged social groups.[2]

How can researchers best inform governments and the public on questions about health and illness? A first step could be to point out differences between the main versions of science and the contrasting kinds of information, analyses and insights that they offer. It would also help to review contradictions between these different versions of science and consider how to resolve them. Opportunities for transformative health-promoting change could also be researched. These are the major themes in this book.

Valid and convincing research

Chinese doctors, Professor Huang and colleagues, urgently warned in the *Lancet* in January 2020 that COVID-19 would cause a pandemic.[3] The editor of the *Lancet*, Richard Horton,[4] pointed out 'a national scandal' in contradictions between two reactions to the challenge of COVID-19. The World Health Organization urged all governments immediately to prevent cross-infection, to 'test, test, test' and to identify and isolate infected contacts. However, UK experts and politicians delayed their responses. Their initial plan to create 'herd immunity', instead of working to suppress and prevent cross-infection, was predicted as likely to cause hundreds of thousands of deaths in Britain alone.[5] Many people knew at once that herd immunity is built by vaccinations, which did not yet exist. It is not built by exposing everyone to disease and to many deaths, a cull mainly of the old, weak and poor, intended to leave a herd of sufficiently immune survivors.[6] One researcher concluded: 'The evidence was not conflicted, it was clear: the Government's strategy of delaying the peak and inducing herd immunity was unscientific, unfeasible and dangerous.'[7]

I began this book in July 2019 and wrote quite long sections to justify some ideas that used to be widely questioned. Then the COVID-19 pandemic arrived and made these ideas about social reality seem more obvious. Six of them are therefore simply presented here.

1. Health and illness affect every interrelated aspect of all our lives.
2. Many causal influences on health are unseen by the naked eye (such as viruses or the neglect of hygiene) but may be seen in their immense global effects on health and illness.
3. The effects are very varied and partly unpredictable.
4. Health is a process, daily affected by healthy or unhealthy contexts, policies, behaviours and beliefs.
5. Policies and decisions related to health and illness research are practical and ethical as well as scientific.
6. They often fail.

Over the past 150 years, research about health and illness has helped to transform healthcare, survival and quality of life for the better, especially mainstream research such as that reviewed by the Cochrane and Campbell Collaborations.[8] Yet a summary of mainstream methods shows how they contradict the above six points. The scientists tend to:

1. isolate and examine each element of health and illness, such as each treatment or method of preventing each specific illness;
2. concentrate on measuring, describing and evaluating empirical (experienced) evidence of the effects but not the unseen causal influences;
3. claim to make accurate predictions;
4. treat health as a product and develop treatments and preventions like commodities, concentrating on individuals rather than their contexts;[9]
5. believe that science can be separate from morality, facts from values; and
6. do little work about why so many research reports fail, when they remain unpublished or are disputed, cannot be replicated, and support inefficient healthcare or at least do not challenge it.[10]

The government and the mass media favour positivist science that examines specimens through microscopes and other technology, conducts randomised trials, constructs predictive models and runs multivariate statistical analyses. These scientists offer pristine objective evidence to inform policy and tend to work in arcane bounded subspecialties.

Or does positivist science do all these things? Microscopic specimens and randomised trials work brilliantly in biochemistry when testing medicines. Models devised to predict the effects of the climate crisis, such as on melting glaciers, are also invaluable. Records of mortality rates inform policymaking. Yet attempts to apply these methods to much social research often fail. Unlike particles, people are complex and unpredictable. They are entangled within interacting social contexts, relationships and needs, which may not be unravelled usefully into separate variables.

Aware of these problems, many researchers prefer a second interpretive version of social science. Their detailed case studies connect individuals' views and experiences to their everyday contexts. This can potentially reveal more about varying responses to the pandemic than yes/no replies to hard science surveys could show, by exploring partly conflicting desires for self-preservation, solidarity and liberty.

Yet some interpretivists are so concerned with subjective viewpoints within local contexts and constructions that they deny there are facts or realities and accept only individuals' views about them. This complicates research about actual bodies, disease and death.

Contradictions between the two version of science and the six pairs of points will be discussed critically throughout this book. Basic new approaches are needed if health and illness research is to be more coordinated, realistic and effective. Critical realism (CR) can assist in this work. Questions remain about why leading scientists and politicians and many journalists and members of the public at first accepted the science about herd immunity. CR promotes habits of critical thinking that can help to increase everyone's scientific and political literacy and judgement.

CR does not introduce or replace research methods, and fine examples of non-CR research using a range of methods will be discussed in this book. My aim is to show how CR theories and concepts help to clarify researchers' views about the methods they are using, or could use, and to extend their analyses.

CR does not look for uniform scientific methods or findings. It works to explain how and why there are differences and why some conclusions are more valid and convincing than others. CR's critical and realistic work responds constantly to each of the above six contradictions. CR helps researchers to:

1. connect each element and treatment of health and illness into many broader interrelated aspects of our lives in the interdependent world;
2. research unseen causal influences and explanations as well as their effects on health and illness;
3. rely less on tracking correlations and making weak predictions;
4. understand health as a process affected by interactions between individuals and their contexts (agents and structures);
5. see how both science and morality affect decisions before, during and after research programmes and how values pervade social and clinical facts; and
6. resolve contradictions and disputes between natural and social scientists, and among social scientists, in order to reduce avoidable failings, promote interdisciplinary research and connect research into effective policies and practices.

These approaches will be explained through the book.

The readers

CR analyses the natural and social sciences,[11] so this book is relevant to the whole range of researchers of health and illness, and related disciplines such as healthcare law, ethics and policy. This book is written for sociologists, anthropologists and health geographers.[12] It is also designed for doctors, nurses, psychologists, physiotherapists, radiographers, public health specialists, care workers and many others who study, research and attend to the combined bodily and social needs of their patients, as well as for interested health service users. CR supports ways for social science research to complement and extend the findings of biomedical and clinical research in many ways. Each chapter will end with questions for readers to discuss, potentially with colleagues in other disciplines.

Aims of this book

This practical handbook grew out of a reading group series for doctoral students. The British-Indian philosopher Roy Bhaskar, with the lawyer philosopher Alan Norrie and the philosopher Mervyn Hartwig, started the group in 2007 at the Institute of Education, now part of University College London. The inspiring meetings were based on reading and interpreting Roy Bhaskar's and Alan Norrie's texts, supported by Hartwig's invaluable dictionary.[13] Students and philosophers from around the world visited and contributed to the free open meetings. Sadly, Roy Bhaskar died in 2014.

Since then, I have convened the meetings and this book is based on the first ten sessions of Bhaskar's course. As I am a research sociologist, not a philosopher, with the help of the students from a wide range of disciplines the form of the meetings has changed. There is now more practical emphasis on how CR can be applied to research. Each meeting includes a doctoral or postdoctoral researcher who summarises the aims, topics and methods of their work and then explains how specific CR concepts have helped to deepen and extend their analysis. Similarly, in this book, the CR concepts will be illustrated by research examples that concentrate on health and illness.

CR is not a version of sociology but a philosophy of the natural and social sciences. It is a tool kit of practical ideas for researchers. CR is not about research methods but about theories and analysis. Whereas researchers are like skilled specialist workers on a building construction site, CR serves the lowly task of the general 'under-labourer'.

The philosopher John Locke believed: 'It is ambition enough to be employed as an under-labourer in clearing the ground a little, and removing some of the rubbish that lies in the way to knowledge.'[14]

In another builders' analogy, the philosopher Mary Midgley compared applied philosophy, which all researchers need to do, to plumbing.[15] Everything seems fine until something goes wrong. Then we need to sort out blocked pipes or floods or hidden leaks. These denote confusions or contradictions in our thinking or flowing ideas that seem to lead nowhere. The critical realist Douglas Porpora contends that there is much good sociology, but it is not as good as it could be unless it is informed by CR. And if researchers' theories are confused or held subconsciously, then they cannot be doing real social science, since science explicitly addresses and clarifies theory.[16] Much CR theory is widely used by non-CR researchers, but studying CR can help them to use the theories more fully and deliberately.

During the reading group sessions, the members talk in pairs and do exercises about their own research and how they have applied, or could apply, CR concepts to their work. The members have shown how CR can apply very broadly within and between a great range of disciplines.[17] They have also shown the value of talking and working through how to apply CR concepts to research, often in response to set questions (see the end of each chapter).

Another key theme will be how to select research theories and methods. Some researchers apply the same ones to most or all of their work. They specialise in questionnaire surveys, randomised controlled trials (RCTs), systematic reviews, in-depth interviews or ethnographic observations. This can be like a carpenter using only a hammer and seeing everything as a nail, a problem that will be considered later. Research method books explain the importance of selecting methods that will most effectively answer the research questions and collecting data to support the conclusions.[18] The choice of theories is also vital.

Examples throughout the book will refer to a wide variety of health-related research disciplines, topics, methods, theories, aims and reports. I have aimed to summarise many of these to assist the general reader while, I hope, not offending the experts in each case. This book is meant to be a resource, with references for readers to follow up if they wish to. My aim is to introduce CR to beginners, or to refresh anyone who has started working on CR and would like some help. Most people find CR very difficult at first. The CR concept of the three levels of reality, for example, is quite simple in some ways but initially it can be confusing. The concept is also complex and can be profoundly and infinitely developed. Confusion may partly arise from the way some CR concepts differ from the beliefs engrained into Western thinking for the past 2,500 years.[19]

CR is often dismissed as too dense and jargon-ridden to be worth reading. Bhaskar's work is challenging. Yet his use of specific terms is not unnecessary jargon because it identifies and clarifies unique concepts in order to understand them in new ways. All disciplines including medicine or law use many specific terms as necessary 'jargon'. I will use complex terms when they uniquely express specific important concepts, and define them in the glossary. Yet my plan is to avoid over-complex, abstract discussion. Growing numbers of CR researchers write very clearly, besides showing how versatile and useful CR concepts can be. Two of Bhaskar's final activities were to take part in interviews with Mervyn Hartwig and Gary Hawke,[20] and in their edited books he often presents his ideas clearly. Bhaskar's 'spiritual turn' is also criticised as confusing, and it is not covered in this book. I will concentrate on basic CR and dialectical CR. There is not yet an introductory, practical, applied, CR handbook for researchers of health and illness, a gap this book is intended to fill.

CR is like a tall ladder, with philosophers at the upper echelons.[21] I aim to help researchers on the first few rungs, so that they gain some experience and confidence. I hope they will then feel ready to read more advanced CR texts and learn about many more CR concepts not covered in this book.

A health warning. Readers who are new to CR are advised not to apply too many CR concepts in their research. It is better to concentrate on thoroughly understanding and using a few concepts at first, and not to use a range perhaps superficially and inaccurately – which unfortunately is easily done.

Health and illness are taken to include physical and mental health and wellbeing. Disabled people and people with learning difficulties are also included, to examine critically their equal access to healthcare and how disabilities are seen as medical or social concerns.

The aims of this book include helping to:

- resolve current contradictions and splits between the main traditions in health research;
- show how CR differs from other approaches to health and illness and what it can add;
- explain practical ways to apply CR to health and illness research;

- guide researchers' initial steps towards understanding and applying CR; and
- encourage readers to become confident and ready to move on to more advanced study of CR.

Summary of the chapters

Chapter 1 considers differences between mainstream research approaches: positivism, a range of interpretive traditions and realist evaluation.[22] The questions they raise will be considered through the book. Their strengths and limitations will be considered, in order to compare them to CR and to see what CR can add. Chapter 2 reviews basic CR concepts, including the three levels of reality, closed and open systems and the possibility of naturalism. Naturalism enables closer collaboration between medical and social, positivist and interpretive, qualitative and quantitative research.

Connections and interactions between structures and agents are examined in Chapter 3. Quantitative research provides vital structural background information about health and healthcare. Yet complex individual agency tends to be missed when the emphasis is on large samples and multivariate analysis. Case studies and other qualitative research with individuals and small groups are often seen as unable to support general conclusions. They are also doubted as potentially misleading if they give little sense of where they stand along a broad spectrum of possible positions. CR analysis of large- and small-scale studies examines underlying realities, seeing how ethnographic and case studies can reliably support generalisations, with caution about conclusions and predictions drawn from quantitative research. Margaret Archer's analysis of structure and agency emphasises interactions, change and resistance to change. Archer explored four detailed ways in which agents draw on social structures and cultural contexts to make sense of their experiences, hopes and identities. Her work offers valuable ways to analyse and evaluate healthcare and health promotion processes.

Chapter 4 questions the centuries-old debates as to whether it is possible for research to be value-free. Can facts be separate from values, as many researchers claim? The critical realist Andrew Sayer contends that social facts are inevitably value-laden and to suppose moral neutrality ignores but cannot remove values.[23] This will be discussed in relation to health and illness, harm and benefit. There will also be reviews of positive and negative power, the relevance and possibility of truth, CR concepts of being serious with theory-practice consistency,[24] and why these concepts matter. Ethics has been partly outsourced from being a topic of social research and reduced into procedures to be checked by ethics review committees and boards. Yet ethics pervades every stage of research, from first plans to final dissemination and impact.[25] Chapter 4 will consider utilitarian ethics, principles, virtue ethics and human rights and also examine the policies and politics of health research through a CR lens.

The aim of many researchers to isolate and examine each element of health and illness was mentioned earlier, and it underlies much vital research. Critical realists also research connections and complexities interacting on many levels. Much research produces huge amounts of data and Chapter 5 presents examples of CR frameworks for organising and analysing the data. Four planes of social being cover all aspects of social life and health: bodies in material relations with nature; interpersonal relations; social structures and inner being, the mental-social-embodied person.[26] The planes relate to health inequality research concerns: material-structural; psycho-social; health behavioural and sometimes genetics analysed through the life course. The four planes and the laminated system are useful for combining clinical and social, qualitative and quantitative research in multitiered analysis. Ways to promote interdisciplinary analysis in many aspects of health and illness will be considered.

Chapter 6 explores processes of transformative change over time through developing sequences. CR theories can assist research about health inequalities and change (or lack of change) over the life course. For this, the CR concepts of absence, change and emergence are relevant, as well as the four-stage dialectic in its benign or malign versions.[27] Dialectic is in Chapter 6, in order to follow the programme of Bhaskar's reading group. Yet dialectic is such a central and major CR concept that some readers may prefer to read Chapter 6 before reading and applying the concepts to Chapters 3 to 5.

The final chapter draws together earlier chapters and shows how CR supports research about the future and about changing the world. It considers how research is always provisional and incomplete, which became especially obvious while this book was being completed in the first stage of the COVID-19 pandemic.

I aim to show how CR assists researchers to be more aware, explicit, judicious and critical in their use of research theories. A wealth of CR concepts, like keys, can open new insights. The final ABCD section – articles, books, commentary and dictionary-glossary – suggests further reading and defines many terms that appear throughout the book.

1

Rethinking theories: the basis of practical research and problems with paradigms

> During a cholera epidemic in the Soho area of London in 1854, Dr John Snow hoped to find the cause of the illness.[1] He mapped the households where the people with cholera lived and tracked their daily life and movements in the area. These centred on a water pump used by poorer families. The pump was next to a workhouse and a brewery that had their own water supplies and where people seemed to be safe from the disease. Snow questioned the dominant view that cholera and malaria ('bad air') are airborne. To test his theory that cholera is waterborne, he had the infectious handle removed from the pump. Numbers of cholera cases quickly fell.
>
> Snow is also renowned for another innovation. He administered chloroform to Queen Victoria while she was having her eighth child, and her doctors at last agreed to grant her wish to be relieved of the pain of childbirth. He helped to transform public attitudes towards anaesthesia as well as to hygiene and public health. Public patronage from aristocratic and wealthy clients was as vital then, to develop and spread new ideas, as research grants and academic journals are today.

John Snow set examples of health and illness research that critical realism (CR) supports. He used three methods. Induction: when he observed many cases and began to form theories about the cause of cholera. Deduction: when he formed his hypothesis that cholera is waterborne and set out to test it through counting households and mapping people's daily movements and habits. Thirdly, he used retroduction:[2] this involves:

- searching beyond evidence for the unseen cause only seen in its effects;
- working out the simplest explanation;
- imagining new possibilities;

- taking seriously a new idea (that most doctors dismissed);
- asking 'what must the world be like for this to occur?' (that disease perhaps spreads through water); and
- rethinking and potentially rejecting older beliefs (about the actual nature of clean water and cross-infection).

Retroduction, a major CR concept, is 'democratic' in that scientists and everyone else in everyday life use it.[3] Snow put his research idea into practice. By having the pump handle removed, he changed the world through helping to reduce and prevent disease and eventually to change medical knowledge and practice. He promoted equality by assisting disadvantaged groups, who had to rely on public water pumps. And his service to the Queen was part of his work to publicise and promote a medical innovation, anaesthesia, so that it might become widely accepted and used.

Many researchers consider they are too practical to need theories or to find time to think about them, apart from as working hypotheses. Yet all research is based on theories. Eugenics was a predominant unquestioned theory in the first half of the twentieth century.[4] Until around 1970, most researchers seemed unaware of how strongly sexism and colonialism shaped their assumptions, language, questions, methods, analyses, findings and conclusions.[5] Their research design almost inevitably 'found' certain groups to be inferior. More valid accurate findings depend on researchers critically rethinking their assumed theories.

Theories include paradigms or the world views that underlie each scientific method. Paradigms involve beliefs about what counts as knowledge and evidence, or cause and effect, why the findings of large-scale research are trusted more than small-scale findings and what human agency is. Paradigms include positivism, interpretivism and critical realism. The most practical way to begin research is to question its intrinsic theories.

This chapter will review: social and biomedical influences through the centuries; positivist health research and the problems with it; interpretive research and some associated problems; seven differences between positivism and interpretivism; realism in realist evaluation (RE); how realism and critical realism are similar and how they differ and combining realism with critical realism and discourse analysis. The chapter ends by questioning the present unhealthy state of health research. This will prepare for future chapters that will show how CR helps to draw on the strengths and overcome the limitations of these paradigms by combining them into larger analyses.

Social and biomedical influences through the centuries

For centuries, medicine was informed by the social study of widely varied cultures of health and illness, by folklore and religious beliefs. Before they could offer reliable cures, doctors' sympathetic yet confident 'bedside manner', their personal relationships with patients, besides their enquiries into the cause of illness, and their cautious support for their patients' and colleagues' preferences were all informed by their skilful observations of social values, habits and relations. These helped doctors to maintain their reputation, their income and social position and their patients' trust.[6]

Medicine began to be transformed from a socially based profession into a more scientifically based one, moving from the study of the individual to the study of the disease, during the nineteenth century. Led by Claude Bernard and others towards objective study and laboratory-based experiments, the movement was furthered when many poorer patients were collected into hospitals and clinics. Doctors could more easily study groups of patients and examine their bodies before and after death.[7] Yet scientific enquiry brought new attention to social contexts in public health and epidemiology as Snow showed.

The transition to modern scientific medicine was slow and painful. Older doctors held on to their ancient paradigm of the four humours inherited from Hippocrates and they opposed newer ideas. Public approval and confidence in medicine grew when effective treatments were gradually developed: vaccines, anaesthesia and antisepsis in the nineteenth century and insulin to treat diabetes in 1921. Penicillin dates from 1928, though it was not widely used until the 1940s and 1950s, and chemotherapy for cancer began in 1946.

However, the main routes towards lengthening lives and improving health were less through treating illness than in preventing it. This was achieved from the late nineteenth century onwards in industrial countries by piped water and sanitation systems, cheaper food and better food hygiene, safer childbirth, less absolute poverty and fewer slums.

Yet these routes contained the seeds of the present rising threats to world health. Longer healthier lives have increased the world population, over seven billion people in 2020 and predicted to increase to nearly ten billion by 2050.[8] Food production has become a global industry run for profit, which involves massive waste and promotes unhealthy diets that increase obesity, heart disease and Type II diabetes.[9] By 2030, 250 million children may be obese, one-fifth of them morbidly obese.[10] Global corporations thrive in the capitalist system of inexorably increasing inequalities, so that one in every eight people is very malnourished.[11] Each year, fewer individuals own greater wealth. In 2020, the world's richest 1 per cent owned more than twice as much wealth as 6.9 billion people.[12] Each year, many more people live in stressful debt. Distribution of wealth correlates with health. Morbidity and mortality rates increase along with poverty, and in less equal societies even richer groups are less healthy.[13]

Rising populations, high consumption and wasteful lifestyles increase greenhouse gas emissions and global heating. These challenge the health of all interdependent species, through the growing incidence and severity of floods, cyclones, heatwaves, fires, droughts, soil erosion, desertification, ocean warming, habitat loss and species extinction. Waste and refuse in rubbish tips, rivers and oceans, with pollution of air, land and water, add to the problems for people and the planet, or rather for the fragile ecosphere of gases, fluids and living species that surrounds the planet. Glaciers are disappearing, and no longer absorb carbon or reflect the heat of sunlight away from the earth or feed the great rivers on which the lives of billions of people and animals depend.[14] Scarcity of fertile land and clean water leads to more violent conflict over who will control them. The key cause of the problems, increase of greenhouse gases and global heating, is unseen, except in its effects. These include increased air pollution. The highest level deemed to be safe by the World Health Organization air quality index is 25. In Delhi, India, the level can rise at times to 500.[15] London air quality regularly reaches toxic levels, when admissions to hospital for heart and lung problems also rise.[16] Absence of water is another hidden contributing causal mechanism. Warfare occurs in highly water-stressed countries, such as in Iraq, Syria and Yemen.[17] Health and illness have to be understood within all these global, physical, social and economic contexts,[18] and CR offers concepts, frameworks and interdisciplinary research approaches to connect them.

Modern medical science is based on a broad consensus of theories about how the body works, the causes and nature of health and illness, and the means of promoting health and of treating and preventing illness. The consensus persists across the numerous subspecialties ranging from anatomy to genetics, epidemiology to oncology, neonatology to geriatrics. The hundreds of thousands of mainstream health research reports published annually work within this internationally endorsed medical paradigm, while developing it in new directions.

In contrast, as mentioned in the Introduction, social research about health and illness is broadly split between two main partly contradictory paradigms or views of the world and of knowledge – positivism and interpretivism. They will now be considered in more detail.

Positivist health research

What are the most useful methods for researching health and illness? Everyone concerned with planning, providing or receiving healthcare gains from factual, evidence-based and rigorously tested research findings. These are essential for promoting high standards and for preventing inefficient, harmful and wasteful services. Valid, reliable research is served by the main healthcare research tradition of positivism.

Positivists apply deductive methods to test hypotheses and research questions through laboratory experiments, trials, surveys and statistical analysis. To positivists, assuring unbiased observation is an important marker of quality in order to increase accuracy and levels of predictability. Positivists also analyse published reports for literature, policy, systematic and synthesised reviews. They collect, analyse and report facts and recognise independent factual realities, though accepting that we can only partly and fallibly (potentially inaccurately) know them. Knowledge is constantly revised and updated. Few researchers describe themselves as positivists, but they accept underlying positivist theories when they measure, test, compare, evaluate and predict.[19]

The rise of evidence-based medicine and the 'gold standard' of randomised controlled trials (RCTs) seemed to promise certainty, particularly on effective interventions to treat disease. Over past decades, they have greatly helped to transform medical care, increase healthy outcomes and longevity, and reduce and prevent illness and suffering. Randomisation is an attempt to construct a partly closed system. Large groups of people are sorted into different treatment groups (research arms) randomly, by chance like the toss of a coin. Randomly allocated groups are surprisingly alike statistically; that is, they divide the large original sample group evenly on all the present known measures (such as age, weight, ethnicity, smokers) and presumably on all the present unknown measures too. All things being equal, the only difference between the large groups is the new treatment given to one arm, tested against older treatments or placebos (dummy treatment) given to the other arms, or control groups. The closed system of RCTs can assess and compare the effects of each treatment.

RCTs work best when testing biochemistry, the effects of a drug on a disease. Social life is too complex to have closed systems. It exists in open systems where many causal influences converge or conflict. And in social interventions, such as helping people to lose weight, it is impossible to standardise the treatment given. Unlike a drug, a weight-loss programme depends on how expert or inefficient each course leader is and how they relate to each participant.

A review of qualitative research reports found that adults on weight-reducing courses believed that personal supportive relationships with course leaders and other group members could have more effect than the course content or goal-setting.[20] All behaviour-modifying programmes from psychoanalysis to cognitive behaviour therapy may be most likely to succeed if the therapist is empathic.[21] This cannot be standardised or easily noticed or measured in quantitative RCTs. Randomisation is meant to remove or even out all secondary influences, such as hope or confidence or course leaders' being more or less skilful, in order to test purely the effect of the intervention. In double blind RCTs, neither doctors nor patients know who is in which research arm, so that no one has the placebo feeling of certainty that the medicine will help them. Placebo can be as therapeutic as the treatment itself.[22] In blinded RCTs, hope, which could 'contaminate' the results, is therefore replaced by uncertainty. However, blinding is less possible with social interventions, such as comparisons of counselling courses, when participants know which version they are having and may discuss it with those having other versions.

Positivist researchers examine repeated correlations between variables or, in the philosopher David Hume's term, 'constant conjunctions'.[23] They check which variables seem to be most closely associated and recurring together. For instance, in long-term health surveys, how do each respondent's diet and weight correlate with their risk of developing Type II diabetes? Researchers run regressions to measure the relations-conjunctions between 'independent variables' (the input or cause) and 'dependent variables' (the output or effect). Regressions are used to make predictions and forecasts by showing how likely effects are to follow causes.

The guiding principle is the supposedly inevitable 'covering law': if A occurs then B will follow. Another version of the covering law is counterfactuals: If A does not occur, neither will B. A typical covering law is that when a dry match is struck and surrounded by oxygen a flame will light up. The counterfactual is that if the match is not struck, the flame will not light.

Some positivists believe that when there is a range of variables, such as lifestyles about diet and exercise, if they connect them all:

> one might hope to achieve a completely closed deductive theoretical system, in which there would be a minimal set of proposition taken as axioms, from which all other propositions could be deduced by purely mathematical or logical reasoning [with] the completely closed deductive system as an ideal.[24]

This was written at a time of 'physics envy', when natural and social scientists hoped to find the presumed ideal of a closed, deductive, law-like system and possibly a single cause.[25] Such views influenced the reduction of sociology into tracking law-like empirical propositions, which were equated with theories about causes. Yet clearly, smoking does not lead inevitably to lung cancer, and lung cancer does develop in non-smokers. In the social world, the covering law never has total results. It is therefore analysed by how likely things are to occur, for their statistical probabilities, when large samples are needed to support general conclusions.

While many trials show strong correlations, others support questionable claims. An example is a follow-up study of children aged 11 years to assess the long-term effects on their health of their under-5-years experiences with English preschool Sure Start centres. The researchers concluded: 'There was a 30 per cent fall in hospital admissions for injuries among that group,'[26] and press releases announced a clear cause-effect connection. The researchers claimed, 'We use statistical techniques to robustly estimate the causal impact that Sure Start has on children's outcomes.' Yet the measure was only potential access to the centres, not actual use of them. 'This strategy lets us isolate the causal impact of *having access to* Sure Start during the first five years of life on children's later-life health' (my emphasis). 'Having access to' means living in an area with enough Sure Start centres that the child was likely to have attended one. No records of actual attendance were checked. The covering law difference was that six or more years earlier the 'healthier' group had 'one more [Sure Start] centre per thousand children' in the local authority where they lived. This, it was claimed, 'prevents around 5,500 hospitalisations per year'.

The connection seems tenuous. Many other events in their lives might influence hospital admissions of 11-year-olds. Many of them might have moved between different areas during their preschool years. Yet positivists would reply this is not relevant when a significant statistical association can prove a causal connection between variables. It is not clear if the hope of preventing future accidents was a salient reason for providing Sure Start centres.

Problems with positivist health research

Positivist social science provides much essential knowledge about the nature and incidence of health and illness, but it is subject to some criticisms.[27] Large trials and long-term surveys are very expensive. By the time findings are reported, contexts and policies may have changed and the findings may have lost relevance. Predictions based on childhoods from decades ago may not fit today's or tomorrow's childhoods. Contact with respondents is hard to maintain during longer term follow-ups. Assessments may therefore be brought forward but then be too short term to be reliable. People may feel better six weeks after cognitive behaviour sessions but not always months or years later, so premature assessments can be misleading.[28] Assessments may be conducted by potentially biased providers of the service being tested, instead of by independent researchers. The high ideals of positivist research are hard to achieve.

Social science is overly dominated by positivist theories of causality, when associations between variables are taken to be cause-effect explanations. Yet these are correlations between different effects, not causes. Powerful social structures such as class or ethnicity are presented as 'variables' clustered around each person, alongside personal agency, such as each person's reported views and preferences. This can confuse structures with agency and strong influences with weaker ones. Chapter 3 will show why it is vital to avoid doing this.

Positivists' attention to empirical evidence (things that can be experienced through the five senses) prevents them from examining unseen causes. For example, real unseen causes include biochemical reactions between tobacco and lung tissue, people's motives for smoking and persuasive pressures from tobacco companies. To concentrate on the variables, people's actual smoking behaviours and health levels, can only describe and measure effects. It cannot explain why these occur. The Sure Start study researchers discussed earlier are typical in seeming to assume that it is sufficient, when informing policymakers, to show a connection.[29] They do not explain exactly how Sure Start helps children to be healthier. Positivists avoid questions of justice or rights, which to them can seem biased.

There has long been concern that epidemiologists are too concerned with methods and not theories of disease causation and that they over-rely on biomedical individualism. Some researchers stress the biological and others the social production of disease, instead of integrating different causes.[30] Tacit beliefs pass unquestioned in much positivist research, such as that health is best promoted by altering individual behaviours and not economic determinants of illness. This may seem neutral and non-political but is inevitably political and has been criticised as a victim-blaming, toxic narrative.[31] For example, analysis of a longitudinal birth cohort study found that adults aged 45 were more likely to be obese and to have diabetes and high blood pressure if they had become parents before they were aged 23. The researchers noted that poverty-related problems 'may have shaped' the respondents' lives. Yet they concluded:

> Our findings support the theory that the stresses of early parenthood on both men and women accumulate over time, and may be contributing to poorer health in middle age. Policies and public services for the sexual and reproductive health of young adults are critical.[32]

Better health services and economic policies to support this clearly disadvantaged group were not recommended. The advice on 'reproductive health' echoes eugenic policies that manage racial futures by means of 'encouraging or preventing the heredity of desirable and undesirable traits' by promoting or discouraging births.[33] They connect to the long Malthusian tradition that blames, disciplines and criminalises the poor and makes them responsible for their own plight, which has fed into neoliberalism.[34] Like demographics, eugenics developed in the twentieth century as a means towards regulating race across the British Empire. Eugenic values influence broader policies, which follow Malthus's view that prosperous groups deserve their wealth and rightly deprive the feckless poor of the means to enjoy life. This includes: reducing taxes, welfare states and free health services; hoarding wealth in tax havens;[35] the austerity politics that led to 120,000 premature deaths during 2010–20,[36] and many more deaths later, after services to cope with COVID-19 had been reduced; and the 'herd immunity' plan in 2020.[37]

Systematic reviews, coordinated through the online Cochrane Collaboration,[38] have greatly influenced policy and public opinion. Their key value, 'evidence-based', is now an everyday term and policy standard. RCTs, which worked well in biochemical clinical research, have spread into the entire range of education, criminal justice, and social and economic services and interventions, coordinated by the Campbell Collaboration.[39] However, as noted earlier, social RCTs are far harder to conduct and analyse than biomedical ones, given the complex open social systems and conditions they attempt to control.

Positivists are among the first to criticise faulty positivist research rigorously. Many systematic reviewers of published research start with checking hundreds of research reports and reject almost all of them for not meeting the reviewers' criteria.[40] Each systematic review assesses all the selected papers by around six criteria and concludes that very few reports meet the required standards. The reports may not explain the methods clearly enough. The research design and methods may be inadequate, the samples too small, the statistics flawed and results uncertain or negligible. Leading doctors estimate that up to 85 per cent of the millions of published clinical research papers are misleading, worthless or even 'bad'.[41] Medical research worldwide costs over $200 billion annually, but an estimated half of all the research remains unpublished.[42] Most papers lack 'context placement, information gain, pragmatism, patient centeredness, value for money, feasibility, and [or] transparency'.[43] Most projects have not been repeated, and when they are, the results are seldom replicated or the predictions supported.[44] Researchers also report different findings and effects from similar (though not duplicated) interventions. They thereby at least challenge one another's findings if they do not refute them. Many psychology findings are 'buried in bullshit', with great pressures on psychologists to overstate statistical significance, publish unfinished work and avoid attempting to test and replicate colleagues' findings or to publish critical reports.[45] Research into genetics and neuroscience is found to have similar problems.[46] Retraction of papers for fraud or plagiarism is increasing.[47]

Systematic reviews of RCT reports are designed to separate rigorous transparent research reports from inferior ones. They serve a main aim of the Cochrane and Campbell Collaborations: to provide reliable, verified, cumulative evidence of any useless or harmful interventions so that these may be withdrawn.

> Not all research is trustworthy or relevant and even highly cited studies may be challenged or refuted over time. It would be preferable to focus on systematic reviews that bring together research in an explicit and accountable way rather than relying on individual primary research studies … research may be used selectively … to support ideas, positions or actions already taken or decided upon, rather than being a rational basis for making a new policy or practice decision.[48]

Synthesised reviews of many RCTs are seen as superior to direct RCT reports because they can deal with 'the fact that policy interventions often shift in their purpose and meaning'.[49] The reviews concentrate on 'the ability of [an] intervention to support the process of behaviour change … rather than the specifics of the intervention itself'.[50] Systematic reviewers explain their aims and methods clearly and can benefit readers with their expert review of research methods. However, the advice implies that there can be unanimous agreement among all researchers and readers on the research design, content and findings, 'the recommendations and formal guidance' of the chosen papers and the overall review.[51] As pandemic politics showed, this involves value judgements and political positions, to be reviewed in Chapter 4.

Systematic reviews have been criticised. 'Existing models of systematic reviews fall far short of this aspiration' of wholly reliable authoritative overviews.[52] There is no simple evidence-to-practice link. Some of the review standards may be arbitrary and ignore valuable reports. The claim that reviews are emancipatory because related groups such as patients are consulted does not ensure that all the groups involved have equal influence or that they all agree on how services are inadequate or should be reformed see (Chapter 4). Systematic reviews of published papers are locked into the past when the reviewed research has been conducted years and even decades ago about past practices. Insistence on evidence base inhibits forward thinking about new alternatives. Synthesised reviews may distort reports of papers, highlighting minor points and missing major ones to fit them into the reviewers' agenda. Reviewers may not request the consent of the original researchers or their participants in the primary research. Their voices tend to be lost, and they might not all agree with how their data are being used. Researchers whose papers are criticised or rejected by reviewers do not have a right of reply or appeal.

Some positivists believe their work should be objective in terms of being neutral and apolitical. Others think they should critically examine the influences of politics and economics on health.[53] This debate will be considered in Chapter 4.

Interpretive and constructionist research and some associated problems

Current dominant concerns to promote 'what works' and 'evidence-base' favour large-scale quantitative research, although there is growing interest in qualitative research.[54] Yet there is general caution about case studies and other small samples. They tend not to be seen as valid sources of general insights or of causal analysis and could offer misleading findings.

Just as the term 'positivism' has been used to cover a range of approaches, 'interpretivism' here refers to its broad alternative. Interpretivists examine how individuals interpret or socially construct their experiences and attend to perceptions and hermeneutics rather than facts. An image of hermeneutics could be two people interacting in a to-and-fro relationship through which they construct and reconstruct one another. A nurse might treat a patient as helpless and needy or as a victim to be rescued from suffering or as a brave and resilient person. When the patient responds with the suggested behaviour, the pair may keep mutually reinforcing it. Interpretivist research includes constructionism, constructivism, postmodernism, poststructuralism, ethnomethodology and other approaches.

Many interpretivists value *Verstehen*, Weber's respectful understanding of the views held by the individuals and groups being researched. Researchers may see their own values and judgements as relevant, or they may examine these to see how they might illuminate their work or else try to ensure that their values do not influence the findings.[55] Constructionists examine how we construct and reconstruct our experiences of health and illness.[56] A subgroup, of constructionist realists, aims to show how 'the contrasting perspectives and evaluations of medical knowledge are under-determined by … an external reality, while over-determined by social processes'.[57]

Positivist questionnaires designed to measure yes/no responses are less useful than narrative interviews can be when researching complex ambivalent personal views. These may reveal depths that require intricate analysis of how each speaker interprets the world. The facts of the causes, symptoms and treatments of illness, the stark biological realities of morbidity and mortality, matter less in interpretive research than how these are perceived and experienced. The ill-health assemblage is the networks of biological, psychological and socio-cultural relations that surround bodies during ill-health.[58] Fox argued for sociologists to reject the organic body-with-organs as the unit of analysis of health and illness research and replace it with the approach to embodiment influenced by Deleuze and Guattari.[59] He applied three concepts: the body-without-organs, assemblages and territorialisation. He contrasted these with the (factual) biomedicalised body-with-organs in order to explore the shaping of the ill-health assemblage. Whereas positivists consider there is an independent factual reality that can be discovered, interpretivists concentrate on how we perceive, construct, interpret and invent our experiences.

Methods that contribute valuable interpretive studies of health and illness include semi-structured interviews, ethnographic observations, histories and case studies of participants' complex interactions within contexts and processes of change over time. All these methods can complement and enrich findings from quantitative surveys, when 'quantitative forms of knowing may reduce the complexity of human experience in a way that denies its very meaning'.[60] Detailed study of a few people with cystic fibrosis can be 'nested' within, and illuminate, large surveys of hundreds of affected people. The surveys can indicate how typical or unusual the detailed cases may be. The interviews help to resolve contradictions found by surveys, such as people's ambivalent views about when they comply with their doctors' advice or partly reject it.

An example of differences between the paradigms is when positivists include 'trick questions' in their questionnaires, designed to check if all the replies are consistent and 'honest'.[61] If there are contradictions between the replies, these tend to be seen as unreliable and deviating from accurate true accounts. Interpretivists, however, may regard inconsistent replies as a sign of a successful interview. Interviewees often start with the 'public account',[62] saying what they believe will be accepted, wanted or endorsed by their expert interviewer. Gradually, as trust grows, and as interviewees explore their views more deeply and perhaps develop new insights, they may give 'private accounts' to later questions. 'I used to think that, but now I'm beginning to realise that maybe I think this.'

Some interpretivists see the later replies as nearer to the interviewee's genuine or true views,[63] beyond a superficial and potentially misleading public level. If uncritical public accounts are sustained throughout interviews and questionnaires, or are counted as the genuine replies by the researchers, they can be used to support rather than challenge current practices and policies. Interpretive researchers help interviewees to move towards giving private accounts in personal narratives that emerge during informal trusting encounters. Accounts may also seem inconsistent, though be genuine, when interviewees talk of their interactions with different people who have varying views of them and their illness.

Narrative researchers have shown the great value of listening to interviewees developing their deeper insights and of analysing underlying themes in their replies. Mildred Blaxter analysed Scottish women's views on their 'health capital' traced through family histories.[64] She found that illness is easier to talk about than health, like Michael Bury.[65] He showed the importance of narratives for interviewees who try to establish their moral status when coming to terms with their chronic illness. Arthur Frank also found how their narratives help chronically ill people to make sense of their experiences, to repair and create their new self and to make new life maps.[66] These three researchers listened not only to what people said but also to how they said it and how they reconstructed their world. This is valuable information for healthcare professionals who want to understand, assist and influence their patients.

Some interpretivists consider that there is no truth, or that truth cannot be known or assessed, and that each inconsistent reply is valid in its own context. They give equal weight to early replies, which fit discussions between strangers, and to contradictory later replies, which fit more intimate relations developed through the interview. They may support relativist views, which see any general standard of truth as irrelevant and believe there are many contingent truths.[67] Researchers' concern is then with how interviewees present and perform their accounts.[68] The main problems with interpretive research include its sometimes tenuous contact with reality and, in some versions, its denial that reality exists beyond personal perceptions. This limits its relevance for healthcare practitioners, patients and policymakers.

Another problem is barriers to combining interpretive and positivist research. Researchers often combine the paradigms in mixed quantitative and qualitative studies. However, useful multimethod work is held back when researchers in each group criticise the other group. Qualitative researchers contend their work is valuable because they can explore complex questions and go beyond measuring, comparing and evaluating. Quantitative researchers are wary of 'anecdotes' and 'bias' and poor selection of cases to support misleading evidence. They consider their large databases produce more accurate, valid and reliable evidence. Some researchers claim that only their own methods are reliable and worth publishing. In 2016, 76 senior academics protested that the (positivist-based) *British Medical Journal* kept refusing to publish qualitative research because it was seen as 'low priority', 'unlikely to be highly cited', 'lacking practical value' or 'not of interest to our readers'.[69]

An anti-positivist interpretivist text claimed:

> Phenomena can be understood only within the context in which they are studied: findings from one context cannot be generalized from one setting to another … Evaluation data derived from constructivist inquiry have neither special status nor legitimation; they represent simply another construction to be taken into account in the move towards consensus …

> We have argued that no accommodation is possible between positivist and constructivist belief systems as they are now formulated. We do not see any possibility of accommodation if [it] is to occur by having one paradigm overwhelm the other by the sheer power of its arguments or by having the paradigms play complementary roles, or by showing that one is a special case of the other.[70]

Although many health researchers observe a positivism/interpretivism opposition, many others reject what they see as extreme views at either end of the spectrum. Numerous researchers aim to work on a middle ground of moderate versions. Yet to work in either paradigm involves tacitly accepting that paradigm's theories. And researchers who combine, for example, positivist 'objective' surveys with interpretive 'subjective' interviews have to cover over contradictions, which are set out in the next section.

Seven differences between positivism and interpretivism

People with Type I diabetes have episodes of high blood sugar levels when they feel hyper and low blood sugar levels or hypos when they feel weak. Similarly, positivists can be hyper-factual and may treat everything as a strong reliable fact. If ideas cannot be clearly defined, counted and measured, they may be rejected as not worth researching; they might not even exist. In comparison, interpretivists' knowledge may be seen as weak if it is hypo-factual, with the doubt that few if any facts and truths exist at all. Policymakers, journalists and the general public seem to hold this view when they rely only on hard positivist scientists to advise on the pandemic policies.

Positivist approaches in social and natural science research assume seven tenets, which are summarised here. They may be applied to experiments, surveys, tests, evaluations, demographics, statistics, multivariate analysis, medical records and medical imaging such as neuro-scans.[71] They may be represented in the image of the objective, detached scientist examining through a microscope, computer or other technology specific data isolated from the social context.

1. Detached researchers observe objective, self-evident, value-free facts and material that are
2. set apart from their social context, often as separate variables
3. independent, pristine and the same, whoever observes, reports or reads about them

4. having, therefore, essential inherent qualities and
5. stable lasting reality 'out there' in the world so that data – words, numbers, images –exist unchanged across time and space.
6. Social and natural science facts provide general laws, replicable findings and reliable predictions.
7. 'Evidence-based' findings yield self-evident conclusions about causes-effects, to support effective policymaking and problem-solving.

The seven main tenets on which interpretivism is based are summarised next. Here, the image could be two participants, or the researcher and participant, in hermeneutic human interaction with one another and with their complex social backgrounds. Readers will note contradictions between each pair of numbered tenets in the two lists.

1. Researchers see people, objects and events as constructed through negotiated interactions, hermeneutics and perceptions
2. within specific social contexts, cultures and meanings.
3. Phenomena are therefore contingent
4. with few or no essential inherent qualities
5. and no general, lasting, universal reality or truth that transfer intact across time and space.
6. Without fixed realities, it is hard to compare or transfer meaning, to generalise or connect causes to outcomes.
7. Connections between data, conclusions, recommendations and policy seem tenuous.

Later chapters will show how positivism and interpretivism do not need to be opposed. They can complement one another's strengths and limitations when combined within larger concepts of reality. The next sections compare CR with realist evaluation (RE). RE is considered here in some detail because it is widely used in health research. Readers who do not work with RE may wish to move on to the later section on combining paradigms.

Realism or realist evaluation

One paradigm intended to combine the strengths and overcome the weaknesses in the above two main paradigms is realism or realist evaluation. RE is explained on a website and in many publications,[72] and it is used in some systematic and synthesised reviews, considered earlier. RE is often assumed to be like CR, whereas RE and CR differ.[73] This section lists aspects of RE and then notes similarities and differences between RE and CR.

Realist evaluators consider that much positivist and evidence-based research and policy work:

- is too simplistic for complex and varied social interventions, contexts, systems and implementations;
- gives little idea as to why something worked or not in different contexts;
- needs to move beyond measuring and reporting effectiveness when evidence is mixed or conflicting;
- needs to involve the views of all stakeholders; and
- needs a research synthesis method to evaluate complex interventions.[74]

Eight features of RE will be summarised and then these will later be compared with CR.

1.1. RE accepts the 'realistic' factual positivist view of a real external natural and social world that we can discover and know through experiment and observation. Social structures and systems are seen as 'real' because they have real effects. RE also supports constructionist understanding of experience: everything we sense and experience is interpreted through our brain, so that we cannot be certain of the nature of reality. We amass and interpret and know and experience only partly and fallibly, filtered through our language, culture and memories. RE is 'sitting between' positivism and constructivism.[75] Realists may involve a wide range of stakeholders in planning and reviewing their work to ensure their views are considered. Yet RE aims to avoid the relativist tendencies of interpretivism.[76]

1.2. The aim in RE is not simply to show what works (or does not work) but to show what works for whom, when, in which contexts and ways, and why it works. RE is 'a methodological orientation, or a broad logic of inquiry that is grounded in the philosophy of science and social science'.[77] RE reviews are confined into past evidence and the decisions and methods of the earlier primary and secondary researchers whose work is synthesised. This often non-realist work is evaluated and may be 'recast' and reworked into new CMO configurations. CMO stands for how Contexts and Mechanisms interact to affect or generate Outcomes. To show how and why things work in certain ways, there are complex RE methods to examine diversity and complexity in subgroups of interventions and participants.

> Realism sees the human agent as suspended in a wider social reality, encountering experiences, opportunities and resources and interpreting and responding to the social world within particular personal, social, historical and cultural frames. For this reason, different people in different social, cultural and organisational settings respond differently to the same experiences, opportunities and resources. Hence ... a complex intervention aimed at improving health outcomes is likely to have different levels of success with different participants in different contexts—and even in the same context at different times.[78]

RE researchers accept that the social world is in constant flux and change. People are reflexive, make choices and so are unpredictable. RE evaluates healthcare interventions or 'programmes'. When local programmes and contexts are researched, they are 'vulnerable to the intrusion of or invasion by more immediate external contextual conditions' that can overwhelm the programme. Conditions include 'political, population, transportation, administrative, economic or even climatic sources.' There is also 'an almost infinite range' of cultural influences in open systems, which can never 'be fully articulated'. All these limit RE's predictive power. Programmes 'by their nature are inherently fragile'.[79] RE examines complexity by showing 'associations and correlations in data from many types of evaluation' to explore and explain why they occur using qualitative and quantitative data.[80]

> In common with other theory-driven review methods, the realist approach offers the potential for insights that go beyond the narrowly experimental paradigm of the randomized controlled trial. It can do so in relation to complex, complicated or simpler interventions (for example, even a simple intervention, such as a drug, is prescribed, dispensed and taken – or not – in a particular social, cultural and economic context).[81]

So RE aims to evaluate a range of possible problems and varied personal responses through its more detailed and open methods than is usual in positivist research.

1.3. Ray Pawson, the leading realist, considers 'the real starting point of science ... lies in "theory", our ideas on the nature of the problem and on the nature of its solution'.[82] However, by 'theory', realists mainly mean their hypothesis: to show within the CMO framework what the tested programme is expected to do and, in some cases, how it might work. The RE method:

- makes theory explicit on the underlying assumptions about how something works and its expected effects (deduction);
- looks for empirical evidence to support, contradict or modify the theory;
- combines theory and evidence into results to explain CMO interventions;
- informs decision-makers about effectiveness and estimated predictions of risk and expectations if something will work or not; and
- does so by providing rich, detailed, practical understanding of the working of complex interventions.[83]

Yet realists accept that their programmes and theory-based understandings about 'what works for whom, in what contexts, and how' and their reported outcomes work differently in different contexts and through different change mechanisms. They cannot simply be replicated in each context.

1.4. RE aims to solve social problems by examining how interventions can benefit and alter the behaviours of different subgroups of research subjects.[84] Rather than conducting RCTs, RE's secondary analysis of RCTs examines the effects on subgroups within large trials and within synthesised reviews of many RCTs. In CMO theory:

Contexts include spaces and social, geographical and historical settings, with norms, values and interrelationships found in underlying social, cultural, economic or legal contexts. Contexts may also include the RE research programme design and staff. Contexts are the circumstances in which mechanisms can be fired and will operate or be prevented. Each research programme can have multiple mechanisms and contexts.

Mechanisms involve changing the reasoning of research participants, their values, beliefs and attitudes or the logic they apply to a situation, their 'choices and capacities which lead to regular patterns of behaviour'.[85] Mechanisms are the 'entities, processes, or structures which operate in particular contexts to generate outcomes of interest and give rise to causal regularities … a guiding principle across many social and natural science disciplines'.[86] RE programmes work when participants make and sustain new choices within their available resources (information, skills, material resources, support). Mechanisms include programmes and their resources, for example, a weight-reducing course, and how these change the participants' reasoning through the 'choices and the capacities they may derive from group membership' or other resources.

The measured *outcomes* are the changes triggered through the interactions of contexts and mechanisms on participants' reasoning and behaviours. Outcomes indicate whether to 'mount, monitor, modify or mothball a programme'. Programmes produce multiple outcomes, which are examined by testing hypotheses on subgroups. 'Outcomes are not inspected to see if [whole] programmes work, but are analysed to discover if the conjectured mechanism-context theories are confirmed.'[87]

> We find the same combination of agency and structure employed generally across sociological explanation and we thus suppose that the evaluation of social programmes will deploy identical explanatory forms, reaching 'down' to the layers of individual *reasoning* (what is the desirability of the ideas promoted by a program?) and 'up' to the collective *resources* on offer (does the program provide the means for subjects to change their minds?).[88]

RE social programmes and complex interventions may change the micro resources, or opportunities available to participants, and the macro social context, such as legislation. To alter participants' reasoning can mean helping them to want to lose weight and to sustain related changes to their daily life. When realists alter the context of opportunities to trigger the mechanisms of change, there will be both intended and unintended outcomes.

1.5. Realists use positivist covering law. Semi-closed systems, contexts and programmes are constructed to test if they work more or less well through different mechanisms or contexts or with different groups of people. By tracing more diverse and detailed conjunctions than RCTs and evaluations usually do, RE aims to show 'the success, failure or mixed fortunes of complex interventions'.[89]

The aim is also to show why changes occur. RE 'always has explanatory ambitions. It assumes that programme effectiveness will always be partial and conditional and seeks to improve understanding of the key contributions and caveats.'[90] Realists assess patients' or professionals' behaviours before, during and after trial interventions and compare CMO configurations within programmes. Stakeholders' views on how well programmes work are collected through interviews, focus groups, questionnaires and the DELPHI method.[91] Their views help to refute or refine theories about how and for whom each programme 'works'.[92] Given the multiple CMOs and interactions between them, as noted earlier the findings are not replicable but they can be transferable. They might work 'more or less well' with certain groups and contexts, at certain times, and even differently within the same context.[93]

1.6. Auguste Comte, the founder of positivist sociology, promoted research to discover and explain covering laws in order to predict, and to predict in order to control society.[94] Durkheim and Parsons developed this functionalist tradition, the view that whole societies function for the greater good. Like other 'what works' research programmes, RE aims to show ways to organise and improve the effective functioning of healthcare and social systems.

1.7. Realists aim to be objective and value-neutral, to concentrate on facts and exclude values.[95] They mainly work on altering individuals' observable behaviours, rather than addressing unseen structural influences on ill-health such as poverty or air pollution. This risks blaming unhealthy victims instead of pathologising policies. RE began with criminology and programmes to reform offenders.[96] While overall outcomes of an evaluated programme did not show big gains, evaluations of certain interventions with certain subgroups of prisoners within the programme showed better outcomes. This led to RE's more complex versions of analysing research trials. The model of reforming prisoners to reduce crime transferred to the model of altering patients' behaviours to reduce illness. This fits the structural functionalist tradition,[97] where illness is a form of deviance and patients should adopt the sick role, comply with treatment and strive to recover.

1.8. The huge amounts of extra data generated by RE analysis of subgroups can be confusing unless they are very well organised and explained. Realists admit that RE 'can be difficult to codify and requires considerable researcher reflection and creativity. As such there is often confusion when operationalising the method in practice.'[98] Research may 'become bogged down in finely detailed lists [of Cs, Ms and Os and fail] to produce a coherent explanation of how these … were linked or related (or not) to each other'.[99] RE researchers regret that their reports need to be longer than the 3,000–4,000 word total set by most academic journals.

How realism and critical realism are similar and how they differ

This section comments on the eight points and raises ideas to be developed in later chapters.

2.1. RE and CR share the theories noted in 1.1.

2.2. RE and CR share caution about researchers' limited ability to make general predictions, given complex societies, choice-making individuals and open systems. RE examines empirical evidence of past events. CR is interested also in the present, the future and unseen influences.

Although realists claim to show *why* things work, they examine effects in empirical correlations but not unseen real causal mechanisms.[100] RE merges causes and effects in timeless multivariate analysis. 'Realists shun the successionist [sequenced through time] view of causation as a relationship between discrete events.'[101] They see 'causal powers' embedded timelessly 'in social relations and organisational structures which they form'.

Yet timing is vital in CR to understand causes that precede effects and also to track processes of transformative change. For example, unseen chemicals in traffic emissions precede the 'new tobacco' of toxic air,[102] which increases children's breathing problems and weight gain.[103] Should RE studies of how walking to school might affect childhood obesity extend to also examining air quality and its effects?[104] CR considers these kinds of political and potentially global influences, which are beyond RE's controlled CMOs.

2.3. By 'theory', realists mainly mean their CMO hypothesis, and they are primarily concerned with methodology. Pawson criticised CR's 'totalizing ontology, its arrogant epistemology and its naive methodology',[105] but CR does not have a methodology. CR is primarily concerned with theories, philosophical questions, concepts and frameworks of analysis, though it can be combined with methods including RCTs, systematic reviews and evaluations.[106]

2.4. RE and CR both examine how agents interact with social contexts and structures in qualitative and quantitative research, but they do so in different ways. RE mechanisms merge the resources of structures with the reasoning of agents, and conflate agency and structure into people's thoughts.[107] CMO is criticised for being unclear about when context and mechanism refer to structure or to agency.

Which has an empirical basis and which has a theoretical basis? How do socio-economic structures fit into CMO?[108] How can advice that researchers should theorise links between variables work 'if one variable is of a different epistemological nature to the other two'?[109] Another confusion is advice that RE researchers should engage with context in their explanations but also strip out context when they identify a generalisable theory that can be tested in various contexts.[110] Unlike RE, CR clearly distinguishes between inanimate structures and conscious agents. These exist separately but interactively.

RE and CR have different views of reality. Whereas RE works at the empirical and actual levels, Chapter 2 will explain CR's three layers of reality. These are empirical experiences, actual existing things and the third level of unseen real causal mechanisms. In RE, the researchers' programme, such as analysing RCTs about weight-reduction courses, is seen as a real cause. Yet in CR, a research programme is not seen as a real cause 'but an artificial structure of inquiry that seeks to set up a relatively closed system. In itself it does not cause anything, it is a research method.'[111] In CR, it is vital not to confuse the methods with the objects of research, such as the causal law method of analysis with the observed patterns of events. To critical realists, 'the idea that research experiments can produce laws, not simply study them', is as absurd as imagining that 'human beings, in their experimental activity, cause and even change the laws of nature!'[112]

RE includes the programme, which is being managed and tested, among its contexts and mechanisms. This also raises confusion between the research processes-methods and the phenomena being researched. Another complication is when effects of the programme, such as responses to obesity and attempts to reduce it, are treated as if they are causes. RE's attention to actual measurable events and behaviours further diverts attention away from unseen real causes. Critical realists consider that only if the real causal level is understood and addressed can we understand the causes of obesity, or of any problem, and therefore the means of preventing it (Chapter 2).

2.5. Whereas RE constructs semi-closed systems in order to test covering law, CR researches the real world of complex open systems and unpredictable choice-making agents. Pawson claims that 'laws of nature are only produced in artificial closed systems'.[113] CR denies there can be closed systems in the complex social and natural world. CR also denies (point 2.4) that closed systems and research programmes can 'produce' laws of nature, which can only be revealed and discovered, not invented.

CR celebrates open systems, whereas RE has a partly negative view of them when they 'subvert or enhance' RE programmes, 'compromise' empirical closure and 'threaten even well-established CMO configurations' so that they may 'suddenly fail'.[114] 'Some have argued that syntheses based on critical realist meta-theory will ensure fuller explanations of social change than can be offered by current [RE] approaches to meta-analysis as these are based on the thin inferences of causality from standard experimental studies.'[115]

Despite the aim of objectivity, RE appears to allow for considerable subjectivity. RE is an 'intellectual craft' that leaves great discretion to the researchers. 'The strength of evaluation depends on the perspicacity of its view of explanation.'[116] If programmes become too complex, the breadth of areas and 'depth' (amount of detail) may need to be cut, in consultation with stakeholders. Influential stakeholders help to increase 'maximal end-user relevance'.[117] Increasing the relevance and usefulness of research is very worthwhile. Yet there are risks to impartial research of involving powerful advisers and working closely with funders, allowing them to alter the research processes, risks not addressed by all realist evaluators.[118]

2.6. RE's functionalist cost-effectiveness, 'what works?' agenda, is strongly supported by funding and policy authorities.[119] The findings help authorities to organise society and promote public health within current power structures. CR, however, follows critical research traditions. These aim to understand and change the world in order to promote justice and equality but are not generally welcomed or funded by authorities. Pawson regards the fundamental division between RE and CR to be 'on the matter of whether social science should primarily be a critical exercise or an empirical science'.[120] However, CR research can be critical, empirical and scientific.

2.7. RE researchers claim to be value-neutral.[121] Pawson believes value-freedom is essential if evaluation science is not to 'abandon analysis for ideology', which he sees as the fundamental error of CR.[122] Being value-neutral can involve attempts to avoid political and moral matters, but CR recognises that all social life is imbued with these matters and values (Chapter 4).[123] As mentioned earlier, values have greater influence over researchers if they remain tacit and unacknowledged. One example is when RE ignores powerful socio-economic influences on health and concentrates on health promotion that attempts to get individuals to address their 'social problems' by changing their beliefs and behaviours.[124] Critical realists are very interested in observing and analysing how individuals' beliefs change (Chapter 3), but they do not try to direct individuals as RE does.[125] Instead, CR concepts of health promotion include changing structures to advance justice and human flourishing generally.[126] Although RE researchers would reject this as too political, their close ties to government raise political questions. They seem to endorse, or at least not challenge, government austerity and healthcare policies, despite the many ways in which these damage public health and wellbeing.

Caution is needed in RE health research to avoid echoing RE's origins in criminology and deviance.[127] These risk pathologising and blaming health service users as if they are deviant, and there is a risk of endorsing the merging of medical and police roles.[128] Doctors increasingly have to certify access to paid sick leave and other benefits, disability payments and food banks and to check that non-citizens are denied free care. RE's term 'stakeholders' misleadingly implies that everyone involved has equal power, an equal 'stake', and shared common interests. CR, however, critically researches inequalities and conflicts of interests.

2.8. RE and CR can both be complex and often need to be explained in longer papers than are accepted by most academic journals. On differences between RE and CR, Hinds and Dickson conclude:

> the configuration C+M=O confuses researchers since it does not separate out the empirical, actual and real [the three CR levels of reality] clearly enough so that they can engage in the iterative and retroductive theorising that should take place between the different levels. We argue, therefore, that the shared methods of orthodox reviews and realist reviews confuse researchers into believing that a realist review is just another way of adding things up. We think that critical realism offers greater opportunities for genuinely trans-disciplinary explorations of social change that fully exploit its philosophy.[129]

Combining paradigms

Since CR is about theories, it works with a range of methods across positivism and interpretivism, to clarify them, fill in gaps and extend analysis. Instead of splitting different and opposing ideas into dichotomies, CR tends to draw them together into interacting dialectic. Dialectic is considered in Chapter 6, but meanwhile Example 1.1 combines RE, CR and dialectical theory of discourse to show the importance of recognising policies and values in community care research.

Example 1.1: Combining paradigms: an evaluation of a community-based integrated care service

Hannah Kendrick, University of Essex, UK

I found applying critical realist principles useful within my case study for connecting micro-level practices of managers and frontline staff with wider political and economic discourses. By integrating principles from realist evaluation with dialectical theory of discourse,[130] I could show how assumptions and problems within the policy discourse of integrated care worked through discursive and non-discursive mechanisms. Beyond the levels of the actual and the empirical, I gained an understanding of how political factors at the level of the real were working dialectically with the contexts, mechanisms and outcomes normally explored through RE.

My PhD sponsor required me to evaluate the community-based integrated care service.[131] Initially, rather than simply try to evaluate impact with an RCT, I planned to do a realist evaluation,[132] due to its focus on how, for whom and under what circumstances interventions create change. Realist evaluation was also cited as being useful to policymakers and being equipped to deal with the complexity of healthcare interventions.[133] However, during the first phase of research, I observed that the initial programme theories were normative assumptions about patient responsibility and the reduction of service use, without much reference to austerity and the political factors that were influencing this drive. Local policy implementers were also constructing certain actors within the service as 'problem contexts' to be overcome. They included 'resistant' patients who were too dependent on services, 'self-serving' staff who were resistant to generic working and nurses who were described as not being very 'good' at case management and self-management. I was left wondering what sort of work do the initial programme theories do if policymakers and implementers obscure political motivations within health service change or construct certain groups as 'problem contexts' to serve political aims? In what ways does this drive certain political agendas, with negative effects for those affected by the policy intervention, such as patients and health staff?

Chouliaraki and Fairclough's dialectical theory of discourse understands social life to be produced through a range mechanisms working in dialectical relationship with one another.[134] These mechanisms include discourse, material activity, social relations, power and institutions, mental phenomena (beliefs, values and psychological processes). This theory follows the critical realist assumption that each of the elements contributes its own distinctive generative powers to the production of social life. In that sense each mechanism 'internalises' the others without being reducible to any of them. Discourse is therefore a form of power, a mode of formation of beliefs/values/desires, an institution, a mode of social relating and a material practice. Social practice always has a reflexive/ positioned nature to it.

RE would be interested in the mechanisms arising from material activity, social relations (interactions, interrelating and behaviours) and mental phenomena (beliefs, values, desires), but less interested in power and discourse. The benefits of looking at non-discursive processes working in dialectical relationship with discourse are that they highlight how those mechanisms analysed within RE have a reflexive and normative basis that cannot be analysed in a value-neutral or objective manner. Furthermore, the dialectical approach can show through empirical research the consequence of some of the more hidden political agendas driving service change for those involved in implementation, in their agential responses and lived experience.

My study shows that integrated care policy discourse works in 'empty oppositional status' to wide-ranging and diverse issues within the health service. This allows it to be presented as a policy solution to poor public finances, fragmented and disjointed care, lack of patient decision-making and high demand.[135] The discourse 'irons out' the contradictions, dilemmas and antagonisms of integrated care as a practice in ways that accord with dominant interests.[136] This can reinforce economic austerity with an appearance of government action on poor patient care, fragmentation between services and lack of respect for patient decision-making.

Three empirical examples in my case study demonstrate how contradictions between the drives either to create efficiency savings or to create less fragmented, and more respectful, patient-centred holistic care played out. Local policy implementers' discursive assumptions allowed them to drive through the efficiency savings and worked dialectically with non-discursive mechanisms to mobilise economic austerity and undermine policy rhetoric about the benefits of integrated care.

Firstly, clinical staff decision-making was replaced with an auto-allocation scheduling system for community health visits. With interactional and behaviour mechanisms this increased stress and reduced the ability of clinical staff to treat patients holistically and to coordinate care and integrate with GP practices, but it increased the workload of individual staff. Secondly, nurses were made to be overly paternalistic and patients overly dependent on public services. This happened through managerial resources placing pressure on staff to discharge patients, resulting in conflicts between clinicians and patients and disempowerment for patients. Lastly, the move to a more generic or 'integrated' workforce model was assumed to be an easy common-sense process, which improved the holistic and coordinated nature of patient care. Staff resistant to this workforce model were problematised in terms of their age, their confidence and individual preferences, through top-down managerial practices and inadequate training. Some professionals resigned due to the changes, while those who remained felt very stressed and alienated from their managers. Patients also told me they thought the care remained very disjointed. Therapy assistants with nursing skills filled the resource gap within nursing, but then both nursing and therapy tasks proved largely impractical to perform within one visit. Some said they had not been officially signed off to give nursing care and they did not feel adequately trained.

In summary, the dialectical theory of discourse, which connects powerful, political, hegemonic discourses with realist evaluations, focused on contexts, mechanisms and outcomes at the level of the actual and empirical, allowed for greater explanatory power in determining real change within an integrated care service and connected micro-level practices with integral political factors.

The unhealthy state of social health research?

Malcolm Williams (not a critical realist) criticises social researchers for pursuing disconnected directions, like an orchestra of soloists. All the researchers write, he believes, as if their method is self-sufficient and stand-alone and compensates for the failings of all the others. Williams asks what each method is for 'if not for itself?' He regrets that he cannot see a cohesive 'intellectual division of labour within the social research enterprise'.[137]

There is serious discord, contradiction and disconnection between social research paradigms,[138] instead of a working together in critical coordination. Can and should the contradictions between paradigms be resolved? They split social research in major ways. Rather than mutual learning and exchange, there is too often mutual criticism between health and illness researchers. Yet research is not well served by this division and rivalry. If social researchers criticise one another, how can they expect everyone else to respect and apply their findings? Sociologists were notably missing from the official and independent

Scientific Advisory Group for Emergencies, though fortunately there is Ann Phoenix, professor of psycho-social studies.

Social research is useful when it measures and describes health and illness, the effects of treatment and prevention, and the experiences of all concerned. But that is not sufficient. It is like a doctor dealing only with symptoms (effects), offering paracetamol for pain but not checking if there is a tumour. It can be like researchers watching water pouring through a kitchen ceiling. They map, measure and describe the flood and how people cope with it. Yet they say that they cannot trace the unseen source because that does not count as empirical evidence. Research theories are also needed to find the unseen leaking pipe and see how it can be mended.

The health of nations is enhanced by all medical, nursing and related specialties being united in their underlying paradigm theories of health, illness and effective treatment, as mentioned earlier (though of course they disagree on the details as knowledge develops). The wellbeing of nations could be served far more effectively if social researchers could likewise agree on basic common theories and meanings of truth, validity, knowledge and reality.

Bio-social-economic problems such as health are 'wicked' when they are complex and involve many different perspectives.[139] The critical realist Leigh Price developed this concept to argue that wicked problems should be addressed with strong science and democratic retroduction (defined earlier). This involves everyone, experts and lay people, working out together what the world must be like if we are to promote general wellbeing.[140]

The realist evaluator Pawson criticised CR:

> It is a strategy for lording over complexity rather than analysing it. It is a strategy with no use whatsoever in applied social inquiry. The science of evaluation [RE] starts by recognising that the fate of social policy lies in the real choices of choice makers and its task is to explain the distribution and consequences of those choices rather than to condemn them.[141]

Critical realists do not condemn the choices, but they aim to do much more than explain 'the distribution and consequences'. They aim to:

- resolve related contradictions;
- combine and develop other paradigms (positivism, interpretivism and realism) into larger, more convincing and valid approaches;

- explain as well as describe and measure;
- show how small qualitative studies can give reliable explanations;
- provide frameworks to organise multimethod and interdisciplinary research across the social and life sciences; and
- show healthcare providers and users and policymakers how the research findings are useful and valid.

To convince others involves reaching agreement with them on the truth of evidence. Thomas Kuhn doubted this is possible when he traced the history of science as a series of incompatible paradigms.[142] He argued that 'the truth of a proposition depends on the framework [or paradigm] in which it is asserted'. He believed truth can only be understood and accepted within that paradigm. Yet this would mean everyone who is working in another paradigm could not believe that truth – including statements such as Kuhn's that deny any general truth. When applied to itself Kuhn's statement is self-defeating, like all relativist generalisations.

The following chapters show how to resolve this problem and establish shared common ground to support valid, convincing and useful health and illness research. This should challenge false research evidence, which supports useless treatment, delays better alternatives being introduced and therefore undermines people's health, wellbeing and survival across the world.

I suggest that each social science paradigm is like a jigsaw puzzle. When we try to combine them, it is as if there are hundreds of jigsaw pieces scattered around but no guide to how they can fit together. The next chapters offer a guide, like the picture on the lid of the jigsaw box, although that picture will never be complete.

Questions to write or talk about with a colleague

1. Does your research draw on positivism, realism, interpretivism or another paradigm?
2. Does it combine one or more paradigms? If so, were there difficulties?
3. Can you list the main questions from your research so far that you hope this book will help you with?

After Chapter 7, you will be asked about the main ways in which you think this book has been helpful – or not helpful. So you might conduct an audit of each chapter.

2

Basic critical realist concepts

> [My discovery of the cardiovascular system] is of so novel and unheard-of character that I not only fear injury to myself from the envy of a few, but I tremble lest I have mankind at large for my enemies, so much doth want and custom, that become as another nature, and doctrine once sown and that hath struck deep root, and respect for antiquity, influence all men: still the die is cast, and my trust is in my love of truth, and the candour that inheres in cultivated minds.
>
> William Harvey, 1628[1]

William Harvey's difficulties (which will be discussed later in this chapter), when trying to change theories that had lasted for millennia, relate to critical realism (CR). Partly because CR challenges very long-held theories, it can be emotionally as well as intellectually challenging. It is not easy for researchers to revise their central beliefs and review how they could have analysed their previous projects differently. There is great interest in CR among students and younger researchers, who have much to gain and less to lose by studying CR. Yet their 'demand' for CR teaching and supervision far exceeds the 'supply' from senior academics.[2] Absorbing and adapting to CR concepts and rethinking social science require time and effort, and my aim is to help readers to do this as quickly and easily as possible.

As observed in Chapter 1, contradictions between positivists and interpretivists undermine the hope that sociology can be generally respected, convincing and useful in helping to resolve serious global problems of health and illness. This chapter sets out basic CR concepts to show how they help to resolve these problems. The concepts or themes include: the need to separate ontology (being) from epistemology (thinking); the transitive and intransitive; the semiotic triangle; open and closed systems and demi-regs; the possibility of naturalism; natural necessity or the three levels of reality; an example of the three levels in neonatal research; retroduction; power; time sequencing; political economy; the search for generative mechanisms; dichotomies and policy.

Basic critical realist concepts

Need to separate ontology (being) from epistemology (thinking)

Emphasis on visible tangible evidence follows Plato's edict 2,500 years ago that we should not research 'what is not' or the seemingly absent or invisible. We should concentrate on the present and evident.[3] Since the seventeenth century, modern scientific positivist methods of induction and later deduction have concentrated on empirical (directly experienced) evidence. Yet experience involves not only sensing but also thinking, analysing and making sense of the original things, events and people that have been observed. Positivists tend to overlook this process, and to see the original evidence (the existing, being and doing ontology) that they observe, as not essentially different from their thoughtful observations (their summaries, reports, statistics, images and other epistemology). Real people are reduced into abstract ideas and groupings, accounts, images or statistics. This collapses things into thoughts. Objectivity is a positivist myth that there is no subjective person intervening during the transfer between the objects studied and the scientists' reports.

Interpretivists, including postmodernists, constructionists and poststructuralists, tend to be highly aware of the subjective thinking-analysing process. Yet by assuming that our understanding emerges from our thoughts (epistemology) and by avoiding attention to the original independent reality (ontology), interpretivists also collapse things into thoughts. In the interpretivists' theory of idealism, ideas are central. If views about ontology differ and are disputed, such as about what actually happened at an event, interpretivists concentrate on the differing views but not on the event. They may believe original events are irrelevant to their analysis, or at least can never be certainly proved.[4]

When positivism and interpretivism reduce things into thoughts, ontology into epistemology, they commit the epistemic fallacy: 'the view that statements about being can be reduced to or analysed in terms of statements about knowledge'.[5] However, CR clearly separates our thinking (epistemology) from the independent world of being and doing (ontology), which we can discover but not invent.

It is usual to reduce things into thoughts, and possibly to see more reality in epistemology than in ontology. An actual distant Ebola epidemic, for example, can be a frightening overwhelming collection of scattered examples, whereas maps and statistics can seem to bring some reliable order and meaning to the chaos. Coloured neuro-scans may be taken to be accurate realistic images of brain processes, rather than highly programmed digital representations. Table 2.1 shows some other common examples.

Table 2.1: Reducing ontology into epistemology

Ontology	Related epistemology
Beating hearts	Heart monitor readings
Extreme mental distress	Psychiatric diagnosis
Food, meals	Diets, menus
Illness, disease	Morbidity statistics
Cause of death	Record on death certificate
Fetus	Fetal scan images
Clean safe water	Public health standards
Practices	Policies
Chemotherapy	Personal account of having chemotherapy

In neonatal units, doctors may attend to the epistemology of the bleeping monitor screens above the cots, whereas parents gaze at their baby and deeply understand the real human and social contexts of the baby within the family (see the example of neonatal research discussed later in the chapter).[6]

Transitive and intransitive

Our transitive perceptions in our thinking and memories keep changing. Yet the separate independent ontology, the being and doing in the world that we can only partly know, is intransitive. For example, it is intransitive and unalterable that a certain number of people met at a certain time and place, such as in a specific cancer ward, whereas their transitive memories of the occasion will all be different and fading. The unalterable intransitive reality includes the actual people and things that existed in the rooms, the specific cancers treated, the structures of the hospital, and the actual local and national cancer services. Intransitive phenomena and transitive perceptions interact but are irreducible (cannot be reduced into one another). During a zoom meeting, no one can even be sure the images they are seeing are 'really' of the person speaking. Yet the interchange of comments is fixed intransitively in time, although through digital technology.[7] The intransitive nature of the past is shown by enquiries into incidents, such as a former patient being given the wrong medication five years earlier. Memories and reports of the event may differ, and the enquiry might arrive at the wrong conclusion, but this does not alter the intransitive event that once occurred. Present and future rules, structures and events may seem intransitive but can become changeable and transitive,[8] such as glaciers disappearing through global heating.

The semiotic triangle

Semiotics recognises: 1) the signified, the idea that is referred to, such as the concept of a person and 2) the sign or signifier or symbol, which communicates meaning through words, images or metaphors that refer to the concept of the person.[9] An example of a sign is a rash that denotes a diagnosis. Signs are communicated through any of the five senses. In CR terms, semiotics is flat and two dimensional when it is confined to signified concepts and signifiers-signs and when they are both about ideas not realities. CR overcomes this epistemic fallacy by including a third dimension. Bhaskar proposed the semiotic triangle with 3) the referent, the original, independent, real, intransitive person (or illness) at the third corner;[10] see Figure 2.1.

Semiotics is a version of researchers' tendency to lose touch with the intransitive external reality they are studying, as if it can be confined into the limits of language or signs. Some medical terms when used as signifiers can diminish, pathologise and oppress people: geriatric, hypochondriac, hyperactive. Researchers search for validations when interpretivists check their transitive theories and positivists check their rigorous methods or 'clean' their data. Yet their research may still be detached from reality. For validation, critical realists would return to the ontology of their original referent.

Figure 2.1: The semiotic triangle

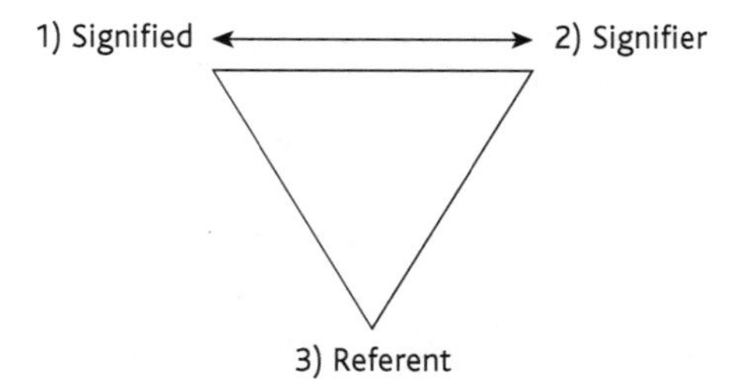

Open and closed systems and demi-regs

Open and closed systems, mentioned in Chapter 1, are another central concept of CR. Closed systems have a single or overriding powerful influence. Open systems have many converging and competing influences. Bhaskar contends that social science involves open systems, whereas closed system experiments and predictions are not possible. 'The social sciences are denied, in principle, decisive test situations for their theories.' In the absence of closed systems, 'criteria for the rational development and replacement of theories in social science must be explanatory and non-predictive'.[11] We search for meanings and causes but not for regular precisely predictable patterns. CR also challenges the assumption that even the natural sciences can rely on, or can construct, truly closed systems. To predict precise weather patterns and rainfall when these are driven by shifting air currents and temperature levels, for example, is impossible.

> For in the absence of spontaneously occurring, and given the impossibility of artificially creating, closed systems, the human sciences must confront the problem of the direct scientific study of phenomena that only ever manifest themselves in open systems – for which the orthodox philosophy of science, with its tacit presupposition of closure, is literally useless.[12]

People tend to be healthier when they have better food, housing, employment and more exercise, but their good health cannot be guaranteed. In social life there is no simple overriding cause-effect connection or inevitable predictable sequence, like the biological sequence when a virus causes a case of measles. And not everyone exposed to the virus and unprotected by vaccination will catch measles; the virus has differing effects on the victims.

Randomised controlled trials, RCTs, attempt to construct a version of a closed system, as noted in Chapter 1, but the effects on trial participants is always varied, never total. CR therefore challenges Hume's concept of consistent constant conjunctions. Nevertheless, CR researchers value and use many of RCT findings, for example, partial connections between poverty and morbidity levels.

The economist and critical realist Tony Lawson criticised crude modelling in economics that assumes total results. He contends that instead of looking for inevitable, universal regularities in mechanisms, we can look for relatively enduring tendencies. He terms them demi-regs or half-regularities. It is 'plausible that there are systemic and identifiable mechanisms in play which social science can uncover'. There can be 'repetition of such a nature, or to such a degree, that an explanation seems to be required'.[13]

Critical realist Peter Næss adds that 'we should differentiate between non-closed systems according to their degree of openness or closure' in the social world. This involves thinking towards more specific probabilities,[14] such as that there is around a 60 per cent chance that B will follow A given certain contexts. This does not mean assuming that when an RCT shows that therapy programme x is 57 per cent more effective than programme y, that will always be the result, replicated in later RCTs. In each RCT, the patients and context will differ. Social RCTs and other research findings therefore need to be seen as demi-regs, with approximate probabilities or tendencies.

Social influences are often dismissed if they do not produce 100 per cent (closed system) results. Exceptions are cited, such as the deprived young people who manage to get into medical school. Their peers may be blamed for not trying hard enough, instead of the exceptions being praised for overcoming great extra barriers. The dismissal implies covering law theory: only if 100 per cent of people are adversely affected will the power of any social influence, such as disadvantage, be recognised. Yet clinical RCT results are still accepted even if they show that a medicine is only 30 per cent effective but is better than all the others. In physics, birds and planes defy gravity, but they are not then assumed to refute it. Similarly, when successful individuals overcome social disadvantage, they do not refute its power.

Demi-regs reveal important contrasts that can inform social science research. Although social reality exists in open systems (subject to many influences), it is still structured through interconnected processes, so that it is not all random or chaotic. There are many orderly patterns although they are partly unpredictable. The reason cancer occurs may be examined through the question why a specific group having a lifestyle x is more likely to develop cancer than the other groups living with lifestyle y. Controlled experiments with partially closed or demi-reg systems can highlight the contrasts in lifestyles.[15] Through demi-regs, CR researchers accept that it is not essential for valid natural or social sciences to attempt to work as if within closed systems. This is significant in the possibility of naturalism, the next concept.

The possibility of naturalism

This section defines some research terms and can seem jargon-laden. Yet it is vital to understand these few terms in order to see how limited much social research is and how it could be far more effective.

Reductionism is the view that positivist methods are best for every kind of research, whatever the subject matter: people and particles are researched through the same methods to discover clear, reliable and predictable findings. This involves behaviourism, which observes and records the behaviours of any animals, from mice to humans. Behaviourism avoids examining human beings' unpredictable agency, their unseen thoughts and motives, or else it reduces them all to crude general reactions, such as selfish individualism or fear. Reductionists guided the 2020 Scientific Advisory Group for Emergencies (SAGE) advice on managing the COVID-19 pandemic. They echoed Durkheim's study of how suicide rates depend on structures such as class and religion. Durkheim denied personal agency and intention to the extent of not defining suicide as 'intentional self-homicide', so his broader definition included accidental deaths. (Fortunately he relied on public records that did respect the correct definition of suicide.)[16]

In contrast, CR involves naturalism when the methods of natural and social research are not seen as uniform or identical but they can still be unified. All the sciences can examine different levels of reality (see the next section) and show how human individuals are powerfully but not wholly influenced by social structures, contexts and habits (Chapter 3).

Many interpretivists avoid naturalism, believing the natural and social sciences differ too much. They assume the social sciences with their mix of constantly changing social relations, freely choosing agents, contingent transient social events, largely invisible social structures, beliefs and values, and hermeneutic interactions between human agents, all require a very different research paradigm: interpretivism.

Bhaskar questions the common view that the natural sciences only work with observed objects and no theories (except hypotheses). This is the empirical model of David Hume (1711–76). In critical reaction to Hume's theories, Immanuel Kant (1724–1804) developed transcendental idealism (theoretical knowledge that transcends/rises above experiences). He recognised that data are not simply observed and collected, as Hume asserted. Data also have to be understood and analysed through our ideas, memories and concepts. Kant contended that transcendent truths are the condition for the possibility of our knowing and verifying experience. Transcendent truths include intuitions about time, space and cause, which bring order, sense and meaning to our understanding. Without them we would only have endless chaotic impressions. Yet Kant's transcendental idealism denied realism and transferred reality into an abstract, ideal realm of thought (the epistemic fallacy). Kant's idealism influences interpretivism-hermeneutics. It implies that social science works with ideas but without independent objects. Bhaskar noted of positivism and interpretivism-hermeneutics:

> the weaknesses of the one position find their antithesis in the strengths of the other. Positivism sustains embryonically adequate concepts of the law (generality), ideology and society; hermeneutics sustains embryonically adequate concepts of subjectivity, meaning and culture.[17]

The solution in CR is to combine these seeming opposites into critical naturalism or transcendental realism, when the ideas and theories and the original real existing objects being studied both matter in research. 'The production of meaning is seen as law-governed but not determined.' (To 'determine' is to wholly control, whereas 'determining' means only partly influencing the effect.) We rely on general social laws, of language, communication and relationship, but our thoughts and actions are not completely controlled by them. Social agents' concept-making is seen as 'both necessary for, and necessitated by, social structures, and [is] subject to critique both for what is presents and what it obscures'.[18]

The study of health and illness in social science involves abstract concepts and hermeneutic interactions but cannot be reduced to either of them. And the phenomena studied, social or natural, are transfactual (they transfer across time and space and so they have partly general and predictable features and effects). Routines of nursing care, for example, vary around the world but also have common features and intentions under any conditions. Transfactual laws, powers and causal mechanisms work across both closed and open systems in the natural and social sciences. Examples include the invisible powers of gravity or of social class, which can only be seen in the causal effects and tendencies they generate. The effects may be seen or unseen, continuous or intermittent, and the powers may be latent or active but they continuously exist and cannot be reduced into their effects. Social and health disadvantages are correlated, but with competing causal powers in open systems (social, economic, political, genetic, space, time) there are always fortunate exceptions that resist but do not refute the dominant influences.

Qualified critical naturalism is not reductionist (it does not treat people and objects as if they are identical) but it can show how events indicate or reveal underlying structures and mechanisms.[19] The social and natural sciences both involve the seen and unseen, transitive and intransitive. Instead of patching over differences between research paradigms, CR shows underlying common ground between them. This helps to avoid interpretivists losing touch with reality and positivists losing awareness of their theories. Another main way in which CR promotes the possibility of naturalism is to respect human agency through open systems and other concepts that apply across the natural and social sciences. They include natural necessity, which is reviewed next.

Natural necessity or the three levels of reality

CR overcomes contradictions between positivist and interpretivist paradigms by showing how neither is sufficient, but they can work together within a larger three-tier analysis of reality. Positivism and interpretivism both respect 1) the *empirical* level of trying to understand and analyse reality (also the level of epistemology). Positivism recognises 2) the *actual* level that the world does exist independently of our thoughts (also the level of ontology). And CR adds 3) the third level of *real* unseen causal influences or mechanisms (also the level of ontology).

The third level of the real is vital to answer such questions as 'Can there be blue emeralds?' Quantitative positivists would collect numerous emeralds. Yet that would not find a definitive answer. The definitive method is to examine the molecular structure (causal mechanism) of the emeralds to show why they look green.[20] Another example is Newton's discovery, beyond 1) empirical beliefs and perceptions of falling objects, and 2) the actual objects, their shape, weight and patterns of falling, into 3) the unseen real cause of that motion: gravity; see Table 2.2.

The greatest scientific and medical discoveries do not arise from directly observing and counting but from investigating real causes that are often unseen by normal vision: the beating heart as a pump at the centre of the whole cardiovascular system,[21] microbes and antibiotics, genes, cells and neurons. Instead of simply treating visible empirical symptoms (palliation), doctors routinely search for the often unseen cause and then for the cure or prevention of disease. Knowledge of anatomy and physiology depends on thorough analysis of the body. Like gravity, evolution is Darwin's causal mechanism theory to explain

Table 2.2: Natural necessity in physics

Empirical	Impressions and images of many falling objects
Actual	Specific numbers of objects fall in regular or irregular patterns or constant conjunctions (Might the patterns reveal the cause of the falling?)
Real	Causal mechanisms are shown in their effects: gravity is the unseen causal mechanism

how species have developed through natural selection. Contrary to the closed system view, the unseen cause of evolution appears in infinitely varied species.

A single illness or disability can also affect people in many different ways at actual and empirical levels, physically, mentally and socially. Social science can be most useful when it investigates how health and illness are affected by unseen social generative mechanisms.[22] This rather clunky phrase denotes powerful social or natural influences, determining but not determinist because they are multiple and exist in open systems of countless interacting mechanisms. They include, for example, inequality and poverty, commercial promotion of unhealthy lifestyles, policies that increase or reduce air pollution. All three levels (empirical, actual and real) are needed in the analysis.

Like naturalism, natural necessity is a common structure of both the natural and social sciences and is useful in research that combines the social and life sciences. Table 2.3 summarises the three levels of reality, or natural necessity, in life science, and Table 2.4 shows the equivalent in social science.

Together, Tables 2.3 and 2.4 support the vital need for adequate research about the 'wicked problems' of diabetes, which combines medical, social, personal and political analysis. Type II diabetes develops in overweight people. It is among the lifestyle or non-communicable diseases, which raise urgent questions about the Big Food and Drinks industries and their advertising and how governments should tax them. The political economy of healthcare is central to the daily experiences of everyone with diabetes whether the health services are free or patients have to pay (see later chapters).

Tables 2.3 and 2.4 are shown in the order in which we usually become aware: empirically sensing and experiencing, for example, feeling ill; taking notice of the actual symptoms as events that affect daily life and then thirdly searching for the hidden causes, such as a virus or hormone, in order to find a possible remedy.

Table 2.3: Natural necessity or the three levels of reality in life science: endocrinology

Empirical	People with Type I diabetes have episodes of hypers when they feel hyperactive and hypos when they feel weak and faint.
Actual	Their blood sugar levels rise during hypers and fall during hypos.
Real	Causal mechanisms shown in their effects: the pancreas fails to secrete the hormone insulin, which turns sugar into energy; injections of insulin are needed to control blood sugar levels and reduce the risks of serious complications.

Table 2.4: Natural necessity or the three levels of reality in social science: diabetes

Empirical	Interviews and surveys about the views and experiences of people with diabetes, their families and healthcare professionals
Actual	Observations of their daily life, interactions and events and the effects of the diabetes; records of numbers of people affected and their healthcare needs and services; costs of diabetes care
Real	Causal mechanisms shown in their effects: how the daily life of people with diabetes is influenced by their class, ethnicity, gender, age, income, friendships, type of healthcare services and their decisions

The rows in Table 2.5 show the original order in which matters occur: causal mechanisms come first when the illness begins and grows; actual things or events occur next in the developing symptoms and thirdly we experience and respond to the symptoms. Yet there is also interaction across time between the levels, such as when actual medication can reduce or stop the cause of infection or when neglect increases its severity.

Table 2.5: Natural necessity: real, actual and empirical

		Real	Actual	Empirical
↕	Causal mechanisms	✓		
↕	Events	✓	✓	
↕	Experiences	✓	✓	✓

Source: Adapted from R. Bhaskar, 2016: 7

Columns in Table 2.5 show how the empirical (interpretive paradigm) is confined to views and experiences, the actual (positivist paradigm) includes events and the real (critical realism) recognises realties at all three levels. Experiences and events are also real when they cause effects. Causal influences may be latent or their effects may pass unnoticed. For example, people in contact with viruses may be resistant, or immune, or protected, or they may have such a slight illness they hardly notice it. Yet the viruses can still potentially spread illness powerfully. Causal mechanisms should therefore be analysed

> as tendencies of things. They may be possessed unexercised and exercised unrealized, just as they may of course be realized unperceived (or undetected) by people. Thus in citing a law one is referring to the transfactual activity of

> mechanisms, that is, to their activity as such, not making a claim about the actual outcome (which will in general be co-determined by the activity of other mechanisms).[23]

Three-tier depth natural necessity differs from flat actualism (positivists stay mainly at level 2),[24] just as researching the depths of the ocean differs from looking only at the surface. Flat actualism sets aside many aspects of health and illness that CR reveals. Chapter 1 reviewed multivariate analysis, another form of over-reliance on flat actualism. This overlooks unseen underlying causes and mistakenly searches for causes in evident, actual, constant conjunctions and correlations that occur between the effects of unseen causes.[25]

Another powerful aspect of causal mechanisms, recognised in CR, is that people's reasons, motives, decisions, hopes and intentions can be real causal influences with effects and outcomes.[26] You are reading this page because you want to learn about CR, or to criticise it, or from other motives. CR health and illness researchers treat observed or reported personal reasons as powerful causes like genes or hormones. For example, care of children with Type I diabetes, who need two or more injections of insulin daily and have to control their diet, is influenced by their healthcare knowledge, their routines and their informed beliefs and motives.[27] 'Insulin is the key that turns sugar into energy', a four-year-old explained, and she often did her own injections. Teenagers tend to become less 'compliant' and often have erratic blood sugar levels. They are influenced by conflicting cultural pressures: to keep to the advised high clinical standards of diabetes care or to keep up their social hopes of being 'just like my friends', 'being normal', 'just getting on with life'. Effective care involves prescribing the best treatments and also respectfully helping young people with their social dilemmas.

In CR's natural necessity, positivism and interpretivism can work together in a greater whole. By recognising unity, though not uniformity, between the social and life sciences, CR enables closer collaboration between medical and social, positivist and interpretive, qualitative and quantitative researchers and thereby helps to promote more broadly valid and convincing healthcare research.

Example 2.1 illustrates how natural necessity is useful when analysing health research data and how experiences and events are real in that they can cause effects. The example also challenges the positivist belief that valid evidence has to involve numerous examples and not a single case study.

Example 2.1: Three levels of reality in neonatal units

Rosa Mendizabal-Espinosa, University College London, UK

I found critical realism's three levels of reality useful when I studied daily routines in two neonatal intensive care units (NICUs) in Mexico. I wanted to see how parents were involved in their babies' care.[28] I had worked in a London NICU with very high standards of hygiene, to prevent cross-infection between the babies. There were also unusually high levels of care for the babies' wellbeing: low lighting, low noise levels, womb-like fabric nests to swaddle the babies, encouragement of breastfeeding, and anxious parents were supported and encouraged to touch and hold their babies.[29]

In Europe, parents used to be banned from babies' and children's wards for fear that they increased rates of infection. Slowly the policy changed, after research showed that when children are mainly cared for by their own parents, the risk is much lower than when a few nurses care for all the children.[30] Parents are now welcomed into hospitals in many countries.[31] However, 'even where services are well resourced and the principles of family centred care are widely accepted there are gaps between policies and implementation with poor understanding of how to translate research-based recommendations into practice'.[32]

At the empirical level, I found that many staff thought they observed high standards. They knew parent care and breastfeeding benefitted the babies, they insisted that parents wash their hands and wear gowns, mothers had to use breast pumps every three hours and the units followed UNICEF standards by not using bottles when feeding babies.[33] However, many parents were anxious and distressed about the standards of care.

At the actual level, parents were 'allowed to visit' their baby twice daily for half an hour. Nurses gave expressed breast milk to babies by tube, but they discouraged contact between parents and babies. In the public hospitals, they assumed that the parents on low incomes were ignorant and treated them as infection risks. There were no chairs for the parents. Most babies suffered from infections while in the NICUs, and one in four of them died. Like John Snow,[34] I made maps to track infection risks. After they carefully washed their hands in a basin outside the NICU, the parents showed a single movement on their map between the entrance and their baby's cot and back. The map for nurses shows a maze of movements around the NICU, between babies' cots, staff desks and equipment used by many staff. Hands were not always washed between handling babies, and nurses provided almost all the care. While the parents were absent, a priest visited. He was not seen to wash his hands, and his map showed that he went to every cot to anoint each baby with oil in turn.

I could have reported my observations and interviews and the hospital records as evidence of the problems. That would have shown *how* the actual practices contradicted the views of the staff and the recommended standards, and the need for reform. Yet like Snow, I wanted to go further and ask for reasons, to see *why* they did so. CR's real level of causal mechanisms only seen in their effects was useful here.

Powerful political influences included the two-tier public and private health services. Those who depend on the people's healthcare insurance (Seguro Popular) are not respected by the staff. Poor education services and lack of equal opportunities in Mexico, particularly for women and for lower classes, increase the problems, which are compounded by economics. The Seguro Popular is underfunded as are the public hospitals, where there is very high demand for very scarce resources. There are too few nurses to maintain high intensive care standards.[35] Costly NICU equipment is misused and lacks essential technical support services. For example, ventilators must have efficient humidifiers, and when these are broken, dry air is forced into the babies' lungs. Nurses do not have proper meal breaks, so they break hygiene rules when they have to eat in the NICUs.

Cultural systems reinforce all these problems. Along with class and gender prejudices are ethnic discriminations. These are related to skin colour and to centuries of colonial domination over indigenous groups. Ambivalence and old taboos about touching complicate any efforts to nurture intimate parent-baby contact. Health professionals' attitudes to women in labour, when neglect and even violence are not unusual globally,[36] are extended into the NICU. There is indifference to women's needs, no chairs for postpartum mothers and mothers are forced to use breast pumps. Nurses upset the babies by tube feeding them too quickly, instead of patiently helping the mothers to breastfeed them. The UNICEF baby-friendly veto on bottle feeding harms the mothers who cannot produce enough milk and their babies. The doctors dominate over the nurses, who spend most time with families and might have been their advocates. Most of all, the staff do not care for the babies and parents as if they are individuals whose 'worth and dignity' matter.[37] 'They have very different standards in the private hospitals', one doctor commented. All these problems are tacitly given moral authority by sexist hierarchical Roman Catholic traditions.

The three-level analysis makes my research more directly useful for informing policies and improving practices. To stop at two levels would tend to support the view that NICU staff should try harder to achieve higher hygiene and other NICU standards. The third level shows that their agency is informed, guided and restricted by powerful political, economic and cultural real causal mechanisms. These have to be addressed and changed if there is ever to be real progress in the NICU and if the staff are to feel able to change their routines. Years may pass before these changes can be made. Meanwhile, we can begin by publishing papers about the political economy of neonatal care and talking with the staff about how they can be more aware of the pressures and of ways to resist them.

More critical realist concepts

Retroduction

Like Snow, Harvey quoted earlier worked with retroduction that involves transcendence and metatheory. Retroduction transcends or moves beyond (meta) the explicit, or assumed, or obvious, to search for the most basic prior assumption or theory or cause. Harvey developed ideas that he could not easily demonstrate. He used induction and deduction to see that every living body bleeds when cut, and he experimented with tourniquets that turned limbs white. Yet his vivisection experiments to observe beating hearts were unsuited to quantitative research. He analysed as few specimens as possible in great detail to see how they worked.[38] He relied on retroduction through leaps of imagination and metaphor to see the heart as a pump. He asked the key CR question: 'What must the world (or the body system) be like for this to occur?'

Harvey's findings challenged and refuted widely held beliefs. For about 20 years they were dismissed by most physicians, who believed the theories of Galen (second century CE) and Hippocrates (fourth century BCE). Harvey's legacy includes the constant assumption in modern medicine that unquestioned traditions and empirical clinical evidence are not enough. Diagnosis also depends on searching for hidden systems and causes, which might only be seen through microscopes, MRI scans or other technologies. Retroduction moves through five stages, which: describe some pattern of events or phenomena (Hume's positivism); retroduce or imagine possible mechanisms that could account for the pattern; eliminate those mechanisms that do not apply to the case; identify the most likely causal mechanism or structure; and correct earlier findings in the light of the new identification.[39] The sixth stage is always to be ready to retroduce new explanations.

Power

One word, power, is widely used confusingly to describe contradictory concepts and CR uses separate terms. Power1 is creative, supportive, emancipating, fulfilling power. Power2 is destructive, coercive, deceptive power.[40] Steven Lukes analysed three kinds of power2.[41] First, explicit power is obvious and can potentially be resisted. For example, someone locks a door and refuses entry, but this can be challenged. Second, covert power and hidden surveillance are harder to detect or resist. People may be unaware of all the options open to them or who is providing or withholding these. Third, internalised power pervades our 'soul'.[42] We adopt and enforce on ourselves regimes that powerful groups prescribe and we see no alternative, such as in mothers' beliefs and anxieties about their children's daily healthcare.

Foucault's analysis of the rise of medical power and surveillance implies that impersonal power inheres in institutions, systems, routines and relations that function automatically, rather than in individuals.[43] Its inhumanity can make this power seem more inevitable and irrevocable, although all social power is enacted by individuals or groups onto others. Inexorable political and economic governance may be so powerful that it need not be exerted by violence. In Lukes's third form of power, government can be most effective when the dominated groups believe they are freely complying and feel unaware of coercion. Foucault's theories help to explain the power2 surveillance society, the great value of people's personal data to commercial companies, and their interest in buying NHS health records, a uniquely large and comprehensive health database.[44]

Critical realists question who exerts this seemingly anonymous power, why, and whose interests are being served or betrayed. They counter Lukes's and Foucault's concentration on power2 and attend also to the liberating promise of power1, working from illness towards health, from coercion towards freedom[45] (see later chapters).

Time sequencing

Another reason why positivists and realist evaluators fail to show cause-effect sequences is that their variables seem to be simultaneous. CR, however, reveals causes that precede effects with research theories that track sequence and change over time. Epidemiologists Richard Wilkinson and Kate Pickett traced how, among the world's richest nations, in the least equal societies, richer and poorer groups both have worse health than all groups tend to enjoy in more equal societies, even if on average these are lower income nations.[46] They found that unequal societies have higher levels of obesity, mental illness, premature births and deaths, and many other measures across all the social classes.

Searching for a cause, they concluded that poorer health follows stress and raised levels of the hormone cortisol in the blood, which they associated with reduced social equality, security and trust. They based their social theory on biological research that measured cortisol levels in monkeys who felt they were lower status members of their troop. Yet it can be unhelpful to attribute and reduce complex physical and mental health and the politics of social inequalities to reductionist biological and animal research explanations. Wilkinson and Pickett's view has been challenged on biological and sociological grounds.[47]

To be understood, health inequalities need broader causal analysis of the impressive range of data that Wilkinson and Pickett collected. Their variables, including hormone levels, are all effects of prior causes and generative mechanisms. Clare Bambra,[48] not a critical realist but a critical public health expert, noted that the UK (in 2016) spent less per person on healthcare than any other country in Western Europe. The UK and the US have much larger heath inequalities than those in other wealthy countries, although US spending on healthcare is by far the highest in the world. It was projected to be $3.67 trillion in 2018, about 19.5 per cent of the GDP.[49] Yet US morbidity and mortality levels are rising, and in 2019 around 27 million people could not afford to pay for healthcare or health insurance.[50] CR validates and extends this kind of critical research into real, prior, invisible, political and economic causal influences.

Political economy

Political economy was developed by eighteenth-century moral philosophers who studied how wealth is distributed. Longer and healthier lives depend on personal lifestyle and on place. Within and between twenty-first-century British cities and towns mapped by local wards, average age at death can vary by 20 years or more. Earlier death relates to low income, poor housing and local food shops, air polluted spaces, neglected and violent neighbourhoods, stressful low-paid work, and other markers of disadvantage. CR researchers and critical epidemiologists search for causal mechanisms and upstream causes. These include political decisions about tax, state supports and services, and how these are distributed between classes and regions.[51]

From around 1890, public health and longevity in Britain began to improve. Some experts attribute this to better medical and healthcare, others to better public health services. A third group cites political influences, because standards of health began to rise before many of the medical and public health innovations were developed.[52] The vote was extended to more working men. Local councillors were keen to improve their districts. Trade unions fought for better pay and working conditions. The 1867 Factory Act limited the working day for women and children to 10 hours, and state pensions started in 1908. These were among the benefits that are essential to support health and wellbeing.

Critical public health experts examine determinants of health as:

1. clinical (such as hypertension, high blood pressure);
2. proximal (unhealthy lifestyles that raise blood pressure);
3. social (work-related problems, low income, poor services and amenities); and
4. the upstream political economy determinants, influenced by decisions made by politicians and financiers.

Political determinants inevitably increase or reduce financial and health inequalities through employment and wages policies and by taxing or subsidising food and health-related products and amenities (discussed further in Chapters 3 and 5). Nancy Krieger criticised the terms upstream or distal and downstream or proximal, preferring more explicit language about levels, pathways and power.[53]

Support in the search for generative mechanisms

The valuable work by Bambra and colleagues might question the value of CR. Is CR needed when critical epidemiologists work so well without it? One response is that CR concepts relate to common sense and therefore are widely used.[54] Three advantages of CR are that it urges more researchers to search for unseen causal determinants or mechanisms, it helps to analyse, clarify, expand, validate and justify the theories of political economy in social research and it offers a range of further supporting theories and frameworks.

I became interested in CR after 30 years of working on nearly 40 research projects. I became increasingly puzzled about contradictions between positivism and interpretivism and how to resolve them. While studying CR from 2009 onwards, I looked back at my research and saw that I was trying to discover insights that CR would have helped me to analyse more quickly and confidently. For example, my PhD was about parents' consent to children's heart surgery.[55] This involves the extreme ends of factual positivism: the children's actual heart lesions and surgery and their morbidity and mortality. During the 1980s much heart surgery was experimental. In the two London heart units, one in ten of the children died. There were also the extreme ends of interpretivism: the very different views and intense personal experiences and accounts of the parents and practitioners, which needed interpretive analysis.

My main research questions were: Can shocked anxious parents give informed and voluntary consent to their child's heart surgery? Are they too confused and emotional to do so? Can doctors give enough information clearly and accurately to parents? Can there be honest trusting relationships between them?

The newly introduced prenatal ultrasound scans could not detect fetal heart conditions as they do today. The problems were not evident until the babies were born, so that parents would arrive with their newborn baby in need of emergency surgery. Was there time to request their consent? Many doctors saw parents' consent as a hardly necessary formality. Their views might be summarised as: 'Of course the child needs the treatment I prescribe. Parents cannot understand complex cardiology. Parents' consent is a misleading formality that can waste my time and delay urgently needed surgery.'

Most research about consent, apart from legal and philosophical work in the new discipline of bioethics, was by psychologists. They assessed how far patients could recall and recount the information they were given – usually not very well, especially during emergencies. Researchers concentrated on medically informed consent. The epistemic fallacy diverted them from analysing people's voluntary consent or their experiential knowledge that informed their consent or refusal. The first international *Code* for medical research ethics begins, '1. The voluntary consent of the human subject is absolutely essential.'[56] One of my questions was, 'What is voluntariness?'

My first PhD supervisor was an ethnomethodologist, who advised me to ignore whatever information details parents and doctors actually gave me during their interviews. I was to examine the structure, not the content, of interviews, when parents and doctors presented individualistic moral accounts of themselves as good parents or doctors. Yet in this approach, it would be hard to research actual relationships and exchanges of information between people, let alone the unseen volition of coercion or voluntariness. Ironically for a sociology PhD about consent influenced by bioethics, the moral accounts approach is covert unethical research. The researchers cannot explain their methods or request participants' informed consent because, if they did so, few people are likely to agree to take part in such seemingly pointless research. And if they knew what researchers were looking for, participants would be wary of constructing moral accounts. Although it might seem to be interpretive, ethnomethodology was in this case positivist. In mistrust of interviewees' possibly unreliable overtly expressed views, the aim of this method was to obtain data that interviewees were unaware they were giving and so would not 'contaminate'.

Fortunately, I was able to transfer to two Marxist supervisors. One was a feminist and the other was a philosopher, working on how Kant's concept of rational Man unjustly neglects human emotions.[57] They encouraged me to examine both informed and voluntary consent, which I began to see as a process, not an event. The parents had to move through an emotional journey from horrified rejection of proposed surgery ('You cannot slice our baby open!'), to doubt, to growing confidence, trust and conviction in the clinical team, from realising that any other options would certainly end their child's life to accepting surgery as the least unwanted choice and gaining the hope, courage and commitment to give consent. This cannot be wholly intellectual. If they had not been distressed, they would not have understood. Their emotions awakened their changing understanding rather than hindering it. They could not feel without thinking or think without feeling. My postdoctoral research found that children go through the same emotional journey before they can give consent.[58] CR concepts of natural necessity would have greatly helped and extended my initial analysis of voluntariness or coercion (Table 2.6).

Table 2.6: Natural necessity and voluntary consent

Empirical	Medical research and knowledge, people's views and experiences, perceptions, recall, accounts
Actual	Heart defects, tests, equipment, treatments, surgery, bodies, mortality, morbidity, NHS system, funding, law, doctor–parent discussions, consent forms
Real	Doctors' aims to heal, to observe high standards and research new medical skill and knowledge with patients'/parents' consent; parents'/patients' emotional journey, from fear and doubt to trust, hope, confidence, courage and voluntary consent

Dichotomies and dialectics

Positivist and interpretive traditions share frequently assumed dichotomies.[59] Bhaskar identified:

- the perceived factual reality and order of the natural sciences versus the perceived irregular and unpredictable concerns of the social sciences;
- individualism versus collectivism, as if we can either be identified and self-interested or lose our identity and agency in the crowd;
- reified, determinist structures (Durkheim's tradition) versus voluntary agency (Weber's tradition);
- concepts, meaning and language versus the material, law and behaviour;
- positivism versus interpretivism/hermeneutics;
- causes versus reasons;
- mind versus body;
- society versus nature;
- subjective versus objective and
- facts versus values and Hume's edict that we cannot derive an 'is' from an 'ought'.

Further dichotomies have already been mentioned: biomedical/social, individuals/environments and qualitative/quantitative. These dichotomies split the social sciences. On the one hand there are positivists, realists, behaviourists (observe actions but ignore motives), structuralists (overlook individual agents) and functionalists (assume society works for the greater good, be apolitical and promote cost-effectiveness). On the other hand the irrealists deny any reality or that positivism can be relevant to the social sciences.[60] In between is the group that tries to combine positivism and interpretivism (influenced by Weber and Habermas).

Yet many social scientists accept the above-listed dichotomies.[61] They believe that only positivism fits the natural sciences and quantitative social sciences, which aim to inform policy reliably, whereas interpretivism fits qualitative social sciences and is less policy-relevant.

Later chapters will show the advantages of understanding how these dualities work together, as mentioned, through natural necessity and also through dialectics instead of contradictions. Combining structure with agency is considered in Chapter 3, facts with values in Chapter 4 and dialectic as a process of transformative change in Chapter 6.

Policy

Health researchers' difficulties with policy, reviewed earlier, include:

- doubt that small samples can inform policy;
- the interpretivist view that everything is too contingent, relative, transient and slippery for anyone's policy ideas to have general relevance or influence;[62]
- positivists' concentration on correlations although these fail to explain causes or how to correct or prevent them;
- their hope that self-evident policies will emerge or 'flow',[63] and policymakers will draw their own conclusions;[64]
- assumed, unquestioned tacit beliefs, such as that health is best promoted by altering individuals not policies and economics;
- 'value-free' avoidance of health policies of justice and rights and
- funding and support mainly for functionalist research and far less support for research about the radical change needed for genuine health promotion.

The rapid-onset crises of pandemics and the slow-onset crises of global heating make all these problems more obvious and urgent. Critical realists are deeply concerned with working on how to change all of them, as considered in later chapters.

Summary

Why do researchers choose to work in positivist, interpretive or critical realist paradigms? Ted Benton's analysis, *The Philosophical Foundation of the Three Sociologies*, explains researchers' practical and moral preferences.[65] Positivists favour practical research, well-supported by policymakers and funders, concerned to make present policies more efficient and cost-effective.

Interpretivists are interested in complexity and diversity and the moral imperative of other cultures when the 'normal' becomes strange and unfamiliar and the 'abnormal' can function smoothly.[66] Detailed respectful studies of intricate local cultures have helped to promote tolerance and respect for diversity and multiculturalism. This helped to reduce inequalities (of gender, race, ability, class) and improve relationships from local to global levels. Yet there are fewer practical benefits when interpretive researchers aim mainly or solely to understand cultures and not challenge them. They may tolerate oppressions and deny universal values and rights.[67]

Positivists and interpretivists tend to be functionalist and suggest only minor changes.

The third sociology, critical theory, advances the minority view that radical change is urgently needed to promote equality and justice through redistributing control over resources and decisions. CR also draws on positivist and interpretivist methods and findings, though in order to show how and why change is needed.

I convened the annual fortnightly CR evening course from October to March and more students joined each year, 70 in 2019. However, over one half of them soon leave. My teaching could improve, and with the students' help I hope it does so every year. Yet there are other possible reasons why they leave. The course is free, and optional, not compulsory or part of any other course. CR is time-consuming and very hard to understand at first. The students are busy and they wonder how to adapt their PhD research to include CR, and in ways that will convince supervisors who may know little about CR. These are practical and intellectual reasons, but perhaps there are also emotional and loyalty reasons. CR challenges many basic ideas and mainstream research paradigms and alliances in complex ways,[68] which many people might not see as wise or worth their time or effort.

Crises such as COVID-19 and global heating raise many new critical questions about what is 'normal' and 'right' and 'healthy'. During such confusing times, CR might attract more students and offer practical and moral support to those who wrestle with these questions. CR can help positivists and interpretivists to work more logically and coherently and to be more aware of their theories, even though some of them may be deterred by CR's critical political approaches. Table 2.7 summarises a few of the main themes propounded in the three sociologies,[69] though they partly overlap. Some names, such as Bourdieu and Habermas, do not fit neatly into one column.

Table 2.7: Themes in the three dominant traditions in sociology

	Durkheim 1858–1917	**Weber 1864–1920**	**Marx 1818–83**
Influenced by	Bacon, Hobbes, Hume, Comte	Plato, Kant	Kant, Hegel
Followed by	Parsons Positivists realists	Goffman, Giddens	Frankfurt school, Gramsci, Foucault critical theorists critical realists

(continued)

Table 2.7: Themes in the three dominant traditions in sociology (continued)

	Durkheim 1858–1917	Weber 1864–1920	Marx 1818–83
View of reality	Positivism, facts	Interpretivism, transcendent ideas	Critical transcendental realism
Structure and agency	Strong structures weak agents	Strong agents weak structures	Structure-agency dialectic
Values	Objective value-freedom	*Verstehen*, relative values	Value-laden
Main method and analysis	Measure, evaluate	Describe	Explain
Main aim	Provide evidence base for policy	Add to knowledge	Understand and change the world

CR analysis helps researchers to see where and why they follow certain traditions and the strengths and limitations in each one. The next chapter will consider how CR addresses structure and agency.

Questions to write or talk about with a colleague

1. Divide a page into three and sort the themes, topics, subjects and/or objects of your research into the three sections: empirical, actual and real.
2. Understanding the empirical and actual: What kinds of data are you collecting? How do your perceptions influence data collection? What are the limitations of your empirical data? What can and cannot they tell you about the actual objects of your study? What gets lost or remains invisible?
3. Reaching towards the real: Where can you look for real causes of the phenomena you are studying? How can you explore generative mechanisms?

3

Structure and agency: making connections

> Today, the two leading causes of death, cardiovascular diseases and cancer, are projected to continue to increase over the next generation. Chronic ailments … include alcohol- and drug-related conditions, diabetes, asthma, Alzheimer's, dementia, multiple sclerosis, arthritis, and Parkinson's, among others; and they are on the rise. Mental [chronic] conditions … including depression, addictions, and schizophrenia [and many others] are now the leading causes of disability, hospitalization, long-term use of prescribed pharmaceuticals, and a diminished quality of life … Reports suggest dramatic and continuing rises in chronic childhood disorders … including cancer, arthritis, autism, ADHD, diabetes, asthma, food allergies … Not generally considered curable, chronic diseases become the subject of ongoing 'management', that is, a life within the medical system. It is estimated that up to 50% or more of the world's population has one or more such chronic conditions.[1]

The unsaid questions running through Teeple's (non-critical realism (CR), pre-COVID-19) commentary include: Who is responsible? What is to blame? Is it inadequate individuals who do not choose to keep themselves healthy? Is it natural causes including genetics that overcome those with weaker bodies and minds, less resistant to physical or mental illness? Like many similar publications, the commentary goes on to list global problems in pollution of water, soil, air and food, oil spillage and nuclear waste as causes of illness. There are also socio-economic policies and inequalities, work-related stress and injuries, low pay and poor working conditions. Are global commerce and industry mainly to blame? Big Food, Big Drinks, Big Pharma companies are driven by cost-cutting and profit-led policies that promote unhealthy lifestyles. And where are the means of preventing and treating these diseases? Should they be healthcare and medical systems, self-help, the state government, the market, or civic society and charities?

Teeple continues his important analysis by blaming industry and the economic system.

> Rising rates of ill health are not the result of our behaviour as so many individuals. Planetary pollution, alienated work, and pervasive ill health are the consequences of a particular economic system … It is the nature of capitalism and defended by the power of the state and corporate sector.[2]

One source of hope, healthcare, is seen by Teeple, a Canadian, to enforce further dangerous structures. These involve profitable 'corporations in health insurance, pharmaceutical and medical equipment production, facility construction, and health-management firms' and costly training systems for healthcare staff. Big healthcare businesses are paid to reduce illness, and yet they also profit when they increase public ill-health. Globally, health services tend to be most scarce in areas where they are most needed but least profitable. Millions of deaths occur annually in low- and middle-income countries due to poor quality healthcare and little or no access to care. However, in wealthier countries, thousands die from adverse drug reactions,[3] or clinical errors.[4] There is the lethal opioid epidemic in the US,[5] and in the UK in 2017 over 4,600 patient deaths involved problems with medication, the type of care given and poor infection control.[6]

Teeple pairs the almighty commercial structures with seemingly passive agents who lack real physical ontology. He commented: 'The human is nothing if not a social creation; the physical does not exist separately from the social; they are as one.'[7] Yet people are not simply social creations or constructions. Health and illness research loses meaning when it denies the reality-ontology of individuals' physical bodies, their morbidity and mortality. Research is needed that analyses individuals' social-physical responses to illness.

One problem with the structure/agency dichotomy, shown through the above commentary and noted in Chapter 2, is when individuals in Durkheim's tradition seem helpless, without agency to challenge all-powerful oppressive structures. Hope of remedies therefore seems remote. A second problem is that the market, state and corporate sector can seem wholly dangerous and negative. Passive tolerance of them by individuals then seems mindlessly self-harming. Yet capitalist trade and industry have also brought great benefits including health-promoting innovations. Third, the structure/agency dichotomy overlooks how social and economic structures exist only through the activity of human agents. Most governments depend on their voters and also on politicians and civil servants. Companies rely on workers and customers.

One alternative to overwhelming structures is to see agents who are hardly constrained by structures. This tends towards neoliberal views that hold individuals responsible for maintaining their health and healthcare and blame them for their problems. There is more concern about reforming 'bad apples' than looking at problems in the barrel. An example is the fall in vaccination rates and the worldwide steep rise through 2018 to nearly 10 million cases of measles and 142,000 deaths.[8] Some politicians responded by planning to fine negligent parents.[9] Yet research showed little evidence of systemic hostility to these vaccines among British parents of young children, who had usually had their first dose. Parents reported problems that they did not receive reminder letters or they were asked to attend at inconvenient times in clinics with poor facilities and long waiting times. When health professionals visited the homes of children to give follow-up doses, the uptake rose significantly,[10] showing the importance of checking problems within structures as well as among agents.

Research is more realistic and potentially useful when it examines varied, complex, dialectical interactions, instead of dichotomies, between structures and agents in healthcare. The research can enlarge understanding of the processes of health-giving or health-harming practices, policies and industries through their interdependent interaction with human agents. The research can also explore the related benefits or problems, possible remedies and preferable alternatives.

This chapter continues to summarise different theories and methods in health and illness research in order to compare them to CR and show what CR might add. Positivist, interpretive and postmodern approaches to human agency within structures will be considered. This is followed by sections on: six features of CR; structure, agency and culture; four types of social structures; a comparison of realist evaluation (RE) and CR theories of structure and agency; structure-agency dialectic and Archer's theory of internal conversations. Throughout, the chapter critically considers problems posed for health researchers to see how research theories and methods on structure and agency can serve their work.

Positivist, interpretive and postmodern theories of structure and agency

Positivist versions of agency within structures

Durkheim's and Parsons's positivist tradition assumes strong structures and weak agents.[11] As noted earlier, it is assumed that societies function for the general good (functionalism). Illness is seen as deviance when patients cannot be productive members of society and they should take on the structural sick role. Although it is 'sanctioned deviance', illness disturbs the smooth functioning of society and is policed by doctors. They determine the diagnosis, treatment and recovery when that occurs. The patient's sick role involves social norms when patients: 1) are exempt from their normal social roles, 2) are deemed not to be responsible for their illness and 3) have the sanctioned right to healthcare. In return, the sick person should comply with trying to recover and cooperate with medical help.

Parsons overlooked the problems that arise when people are ill but doctors refuse to confirm this, or when individuals disagree with the doctors' diagnosis, or when they cannot access adequate care, or they cannot recover. These problems especially affect people with long-term illnesses and disabilities who may be in the greatest need, but they do not fit Parsons's model. He also listed an 'illegitimate role' when people have a condition that is stigmatised by others. Disabled people have long campaigned against being classed as sick and stigmatised deviants.[12] In Bourdieu's field and *habitus*, structures also dominate over agents who are set into group cultures, with learned habits and dispositions anchored in the body into which they are socialised.[13]

Positivist economics is dominated by structures around an imagined agent. *Homo economicus* is driven by instrumental self-interest and the power of money. However, McCarraher challenged more than 200 years of post-Enlightenment assumptions about the way we are all supposed to live and work.[14] He railed against 'the ensemble of falsehoods that comprise the foundation of economics', which offer 'a specious portrayal of human beings and a fictional account of their history', a shabby, degrading construct that betrays the truth of human experience and our hope of survival amid ecological destruction.

The health and wellbeing programmes of mindfulness and cognitive behaviour therapy might seem to respect agents' character and integrity. Yet the multibillion-dollar industry has been criticised for being a neoliberal instrument of social control, not of fulfilment.[15] The programmes depoliticise anxiety and distress when they imply that individuals must mistrust and control their emotions instead of understanding them as potentially warning signs of social and political threats. The programmes teach that the problem is not capitalism but individuals' failure to be mindful and resilient in precarious and uncertain economies. The programmes individualise and pathologise painful emotions when they imply that people must contain and subdue them instead of learning through them about the inner stirrings of empathy and solidarity with others who are also oppressed or deprived. Critics of mindfulness say that to promote real wellbeing involves increasing our wellbeing and freedom through creatively managing our inner resources in these ways.

Žižek considers that mindfulness draws people into 'the hegemonic ideology of global capitalism' so that they 'fully participate in the capitalist dynamic while retaining the appearance of mental sanity'.[16] This false notion of sanity adds to pressures on people to conform inwardly and outwardly. It diverts them from political awareness and collective protest, isolating them into a world of individual winners or losers.

The programmes fulfil Bourdieu's warnings that neoliberalism promotes our faith in market forces to increase our social capital, while it destroys collective structures that may impede pure market logic.[17] Mindfulness offers ways to endure toxic systems, rather than to critically question the historical, cultural and political conditions that are responsible for social suffering. Yet when mindfulness draws on its Buddhist origins, it can help to sort out minor anxieties from serious social concerns and to calm the former in order to work on reforming the latter by cultivating critical thinking and judgement.[18]

A main promoter of the happiness industry, the economist Lord Layard, sees happiness as a vague commodity to be measured and marketed.[19] William Davies,[20] a critical though not a CR analyst, reveals the emptiness of a so-called happiness science without a clearly defined subject or meaning. In attempts to fill the deficit of meaning in mindfulness, ideas are imported from Buddhism. Yet that is stripped of its original spiritual and political dimensions, to become an empty inner gaze measured for its monetary value. The happiness industry blames and medicates 'individuals for their own misery and ignores the context that has contributed to it'.[21] Davies traces both the happiness and the surveillance industries back to Bentham,[22] father of pleasure/pain utilitarianism and of the panoptican prison. There, the watchful power2 gaze of the hidden warders observing every cell becomes internalised by the prisoners, analysed by Foucault and Rose (see Chapter 2).[23]

Davies analyses how Western economies depend more and more on people's emotional engagements with their work, consumerism and their health and wellbeing. But there are paradoxical growing social disengagements, through stress and psychosomatic and mental illnesses. These especially increase in the most unequal, materialistic and competitive societies,[24] which mostly depend on workers' emotional commitment when other rewards of fulfilling work, fair pay and good working conditions are missing. Davies contends that the economic model oppresses 'precisely the psychological attributes it depends upon'. The model promotes 'silent relationships to the self, rather than vocal relationships to each other' in critical, democratic, cooperative problem-solving.[25] The happiness industry transforms stress from a political problem into a medical one and precarious work into a personal anxiety. Lucrative therapies and mood-altering technologies are supposed to solve the problems but reinforce pathologising neoliberalism.

Mindfulness is said to help us to be more mentally fit and productive workers, like a gym workout. Yet the privatising and medicalising of stress, and of individuals' duty to find inner contentment and harmony, Mark Fisher contended, have almost destroyed the concept of the public. This depends on shared respect, empathy and solidarity.[26] Wellbeing programmes especially blame and add to the burdens of the most disadvantaged, those with the greatest need of social and political reforms.[27] Claims that mindfulness is a science show the vital need in all the sciences to examine basic theories and assumptions, in this case how structures and agents, politics and economics, blame and responsibility are all defined and understood, as this chapter explores.

CR analysis could add to Davies's insightful work by emphasising how political and economic drivers are generative mechanisms. Although quantitative research that supports the happiness science appears to centre on individuals (agents), it works to defuse and disable their critical rational emotional responses to their personal contexts and potential problem-solving. It reconstructs inner personal emotions of anxiety, depression and happiness as if they are detached, outer, impersonal structures or systems, which individuals should negotiate. The effect can be to fragment personal inner being instead of aiding cohesion and confirming integrity.[28] Mindfulness, its measures and management, adheres to Durkheimian positivism, where claims to objective value-freedom hide strong moral and political norms of functionalism.[29] In order to obtain manageable measures and serve covering law theory,[30] positivist and realist research emphasise impersonal contexts, structures and events. These are analysed as variables, by which to group the numerous anonymous respondents.

Although happiness can only partly be defined, and therefore assessed or measured, many other categories can be measured by positivism clearly and broadly enough to provide essential information for understanding health and illness. They include countless reports on types of illness and treatment, health promotion and illness prevention and their social, political and economic contexts and outcomes. Yet the general theme in quantitative research is of weak agents, classified by their groupings into strongly determining if not determinist variables and structures.

Interpretive versions of agency within structures

Interpretive research ranges from fairly realistic understandings of agency and embodied health and illness,[31] to postmodern agnosticism or denial of bodily reality.[32] This section considers interviews, ethnographies, case studies and grounded theory, all valuable qualitative methods that cover all aspects of health and illness from birth to death.[33] Geertz questioned the idea of an authentic 'true self', a coherent, continuous being: 'we are all wearing masks all the time through all the changes of social morphology'.[34] Following Deleuze and Guattari,[35] disembodiment in postmodern research concentrates on the body-without-organs,[36] as well as on the ill-health assemblage in networks of biological, psychological and socio-cultural relations.

Unlike the positivist view that research mirrors reality, interpretivists 'view data as constructed, not simply out there in the world waiting to be discovered and gathered'. They interpret data through what they see as 'multiple realities'.[37] CR recognises only one layered reality with multiple ways of experiencing and interpreting it, and terms the collapsing of reality-ontology into reflexive experience-epistemology as the epistemic fallacy.

Interpretive research is informed by symbolic interactionism, the theory that words, gestures and other symbols invested with taken-for-granted meanings facilitate communication and other interactions. Erving Goffman's ethnographies of total institutions, such as mental asylums, trace how the staff and patients perform their daily activities, conversations and rituals, and each present a range of selves or persona in response to contexts.[38] Yet in Goffman's work it is not clear if the agents have any inner self that chooses and wears the performed selves or if the agents are solely a series of performances reacting to contexts.

Earlier ethnographies by colonialist anthropologists would not pass today's ethics reviews,[39] when they assumed they need not explain or request consent to their covert, intrusive research. Consent would be counterproductive when it would alter people's 'naturally occurring' activities through making them aware of being observed. Today's ethnographers, usually with consent, examine people's reliance on assumed meanings in their speech and behaviours, and the 'situated' character of their interactions,[40] with interest in observed processes rather than social structures. Ethnography is a rich flexible method, not confined to postmodernism, and can study agency and structure in the political economy and adverse effects on health, for example, of young Black men in the US. 'The sheer scope of policing and imprisonment in poor Black neighborhoods is transforming community life in ways that are deep and enduring, not only for the young men who are their targets but for their family members, partners, and neighbors.'[41]

Interpretive researchers favour grounded theory, which has contributed to much useful health research, and modified grounded theory combines well with CR. Grounded 'theory' refers to researchers' generalisations or inductive hypotheses when they gradually form generalisations, groupings and analytic categories from collected examples.[42] Texts on grounded theory concentrate on methods of sampling, data coding and analysis, in qualitative research that echoes quantitative methods of organising individuals into groups. The fewest possible groups are identified, and 'saturation' is reached when these appear to cover every individual new case. Glaser and Strauss's theory is mainly conclusions drawn from data by working between abstraction and reality and requires four properties:[43]

1. to fit closely to the substantive area in which it will be used;
2. to be readily understandable and make sense to the lay people concerned;
3. to apply generally to many diverse, daily situations within that substantive area; and
4. to allow the user of the theory partial control over the structure and process of that area as it changes through time.

In their research about patients having terminal care, Glaser and Strauss criticised logical deduction, most often used in quantitative research, for tending to be based on too many unquestioned assumptions and selective data and too fixed to fit ever-changing everyday reality.[44] Their own inductive analysis included diverse data from interviews, observations, documents and surveys. They categorised the care of all the patients they observed into 'death expectations', 'nothing more to do', 'lingering' and 'social loss'.

Glaser and Strauss advised researchers to start by collecting data before looking at the related literature. 'A researcher does not begin a project with a preconceived theory in mind.' Instead the researcher 'allows the theory to emerge from the data' when tentative theories are developed into conclusions.[45] This advice has been criticised.[46] Researchers unfamiliar with the related literature risk simply repeating earlier published work. Yet the anthropologists' approach of open-minded initial enquiry in grounded theory is also valued in CR, along with extensive literature reviews that can raise further questions in the early stages of research.[47]

Grounded theory researchers are further advised to conduct open or semi-structured interviews in order to obtain more 'authentic accounts' than questionnaires achieve.[48] 'Insider' researchers who are familiar with the context and the participants benefit from having detailed prior knowledge and potentially easier access, whereas 'outsider' researchers, or strangers, have the advantage that they are more likely to notice, question and analyse ideas that insiders may take for granted and not notice or question.[49] The aim is to 'find reality' within the interview and in life around it. There is analysis of how interviewees repeat familiar cultural tales and other constructions that emerge through symbolic interactions between interviewees and interviewers. Observations and reflexive qualitative interviews can involve stories that allow us to understand and theorise the social world and the cultural forms people use.

Grounded theory researchers have been warned to rely on observed 'naturally occurring data' rather than on constructed though open-ended interviews.[50] But this advice is questioned when, in social data, there is no neat difference between natural and cultural or, in interviews, between local events and underlying external realities. Interpretivists see reality as relative rather than fixed. Truth is 'context specific, invented if you will, to fit the demands of the subjective interactive interview'.[51] Interpretive research is descriptive rather than evaluative. It involves valuable approaches and methods through which to explore structure and agency that CR can develop, as later sections will consider.

Postmodern versions of agency within structures

This section considers varied approaches: social constructivism, ethnomethodology, conversation analysis, critical discourse analysis and actor network theory. Social constructivism tends to reduce the human body into personal perceptions and accounts. Bryan Turner traced the development of social constructivism back to the German thinkers Nietzsche, Gehlen and Berger.[52] He calls their work 'controversial' and 'somewhat paradoxical' because of their associations with Nazism. They proposed that because we cannot constantly reflect on the countless everyday aspects of daily life, we subconsciously construct or project a pragmatic, taken-for-granted, factual but false character onto the social world. David Pilgrim considers, 'Their Continental idealist tradition culminated in the post-truth society and fed the postmodern obsession with epistemology and the scornful abandonment of ontology. We are all suffering the consequences of the mindless "everything is socially constructed" mantra in social science.'[53] Dire effects on health from truth-denying relativist fake news are seen in populist politics that increase mistrust and inequalities, destroy public health services and incite panic, such as in anti-vax campaigns.[54]

Ethnomethodologists claim to be different and separate from sociologists, by classifying individuals' social actions within groups without (they believe) imposing their own opinions about social order.[55] They create accounts of people's methods for negotiating and ordering everyday situations.[56] Their reliance on observed talk and behaviours is reductionist and behaviourist. It avoids objective reality and unseen or external influences, such as individuals' actual body or history, motives or values. This is another claimed difference from sociology.[57] Yet this assumedly neutral detachment is itself a value judgement and can support a lack of empathy. To expose people's illusions of reality, Harold Garfinkel conducted covert ethnomethodology 'degradation' experiments. He suddenly imposed bizarre situations and watched people's confused reactions with methods that have been described as 'cruel'.[58] Ethnomethodologists dismiss the relevance of truth in interviewees' accounts. They examine the method rather than the content of the talk, the rhetorical constructs of moral accounts but not the actual events they describe.[59] For example, parents were invited in their 'moral accounts' to invoke norms and construct 'atrocity stories' about substandard healthcare for their child.[60] When researchers treat the truth and accuracy of people's accounts as irrelevant and implicitly unreliable, they step outside ordinary human relationships that rely on truth as the default.[61] This calls into question the veracity of ethnomethodologists' own reports. Are these also moral accounts and why should their substance be believed?

Conversation analysis (CA) grew out of ethnomethodology,[62] and it takes reality to be constructed, not discovered. CA also takes language and the social organisation of conversation to be the generic topic of investigation. Conversation analysts see mastery of language as central to competent social interaction, which they relate to social class, and associated health status, in agents' degrees of verbal competence. They use 'real-world' transcriptions of recordings for analysis of speech exchanges with all their pauses, hesitations and turn-taking. CA is valuable in analysing how patients can be encouraged to take a greater share in discussions with doctors during medical examinations, the diagnostic stages of the consultation and decision making about treatment.[63]

Moral accounts and CA could potentially usefully deconstruct deceptive discourses of, say, powerful politicians, but they seem to be mainly used on powerless groups. Critical discourse analysis, however, is applied in this useful way to unpick oppressive fallacies, such as when English health and welfare policy reports generally ignore children as persons and reduce the child's mind to the brain, which comes to represent the child. This 'highly reductionist and limiting construction of the child … with its accompanying deterministic perspective on parenting, overlooks children's embodied lives and this has implications for the design of children's health and welfare services'.[64] Another example is Hannah Kendrick's dialectical theory of discourse combined with RE and CR.[65]

Among the many versions of postmodernism is actor network theory (ANT). Like ethnomethodology it is influenced by symbolic interactionism. ANT treats events, relations and meanings as if each is newly formed and constructed as a single network or performance, detached from past events and other realities, which are 'bracketed' off. An example examines doctors' tendency to look only at the part of the body in which they specialise, so that patients with several illnesses can feel almost divided into several parts. A postmodern ethnography treats this experience as if it reflects an actual reality: '… there is no longer a single passive object … instead objects come into being – and disappear … reality multiplies. The body, the patient, the disease, the doctor, the technician, the technology: all of these are more than one.'[66] 'In theory the body may be single but in practice it is multiple because there are many body practices and therefore many bodies.'[67] However, a CR response is that although patients can feel fragmented and there may be more than one disease, doctor, technician and technology, there is still only one body and patient.

ANT treats agency as existing within networks but not outside networks within agents. The insistence on observed interactions, in CR terms, is flat actualism, and it therefore describes but does not explain. Agency, it is claimed in ANT, is dispersed. It 'neither starts nor finishes with any individual agent'. It is orchestrated within narrative structures; character is not 'real' and there is no single author but always multiple authors of agency. Agency is never a property and is always relational, in between, dispersed.[68]

ANT maps relations that are both semiotic (between signs and concepts) and material (between things, bodies, people and machines). Everything animate or inanimate is counted as more or less equal actors or 'actants' within networks. A knife that cuts equates to the surgeon who cuts with it. '[A]ny thing that does modify a state of affairs by making a difference is an actor – or if it has no figuration yet, an actant.'[69] Children on ventilators in intensive care are

> 'quasi-objects' … consisting of both 'soft' human flesh and 'hard' technological artefact … technomorphic. [Children and machines] are so inextricably linked that it is analytically unfruitful to begin with these two categories (human and non-human) as separate explanatory resources … [The difference] is not in principle discernible.[70]

Yet to conflate metal and plastic machines with vulnerable, sentient, beloved and irreplaceable children, able to suffer and to flourish, overlooks human ontology: the living person in the body and within human relationships.[71] It raises moral confusion about the comparative value of a child and a machine. ANT's actors who react to contexts but do so without consciousness, intention or self-awareness have been compared to zombies.[72]

ANT is supposed to provide an analytics that deepens and enriches analysis and is able to explain agency in relation to contingent empirical realities.[73] The aim is to avoid simplistic analysis and to open up problem spaces within which sociologists can analyse, define, interpret and research tactical agency, agency in resistance and compliance, and hybrid in-between agency. However, contrary to ANT, real major illness and treatment highlight each individual's partly bounded, embodied agency, channelled through personal decisions to consent to healthcare treatment or to refuse it. These are topics that ANT authors tend to avoid when they theorise agency as vague and diffuse.[74] They overlook the reality of individuals' embodied agency and human rights, which tend to be ignored or overridden, pathologised or collapsed into the observer's gaze. ANT leaves illnesses without actual bodies and rights without rights-holders.

In postmodern sociology, thin theories become detached from physical reality, from economics and morality. ANT describes *how* but does not explain *why* its claimed networks cohere, work, endure or fail. And when people are theorised as if they are like mindless and motiveless machines, there cannot be a 'why' in terms of conscious personal agency, intentions, choices, decisions, interactions and responses.

Critical realist theories of agency and structure

So far, this chapter has raised strengths and problems in a range of positivist and interpretive concepts of agency and structure. The following sections consider how critical realists aim to offer more coherent and valid insights through: six features of CR; theories of structure, agency and culture, and of social structures. RE and CR theories of structure and agency are compared, followed by structure-agency dialectic and internal conversations.

Six features of critical realism

These six features underlie CR research and researchers' own agency.[75] Some terms are explained in earlier chapters and in the glossary.

1. Under-labouring, a main task of CR, clears away unhelpful misleading ideas in order to promote clear critical thinking.
2. Seriousness relies on theory-practice consistency and common sense,[76] such as in enquiry about how the above theories of agency are confirmed or denied by readers' own personal experiences. Do we feel that we are each a conscious, intentional, embodied, partly unique human being, or not, or only partly? Researchers are inconsistent if they deny individual agency in theory but claim it for themselves in practice. It is inconsistent when researchers, first, treat research participants as dispersed non-centred beings and agency as never a property but always relational and in between but, second, name themselves as authors of their reports and complain about plagiarism. Although authors gather most of their material from others, they (should) use that to create a unique new work. Logical theory-practice consistency, a philosophy to live and act by, with justice and equity between researchers and researched individuals is part of the CR aim to be serious.
3. Immanent critique assesses systems and beliefs from the inside to unravel internal inconsistencies and contradictions.
4. Critical philosophy increases our awareness of our partly subconscious thinking, assumptions and prejudices. It is congruent with daily reality and the one world we live in. It starts with

the question: 'What must the world be like for, say, these forms of agency to occur?' In other paradigms, 'theories' are mainly deliberate hypotheses or concluding generalisations. Useful though these can be, they usually miss the CR concept of theories as world views, explanations, definitions and critical analyses of assumptions.
5. Transformative practice involves developing a more coherent philosophy of social science to give more valid, convincing accounts of the world we study and to connect more closely to policy and practice.
6. Hermeticism keeps checking whether ideas are true and accurate and make sense. It is part of being serious.

Structure, agency and culture

Along with structures and agents, Margaret Archer emphasises the third dimension, culture.[77] Culture is the subjective meaningful context produced through human intentions and hermeneutics. Agents provide and use health services, and structures are the material, political and economic systems. Culture provides the ethos, all the beliefs about what health and illness mean and how we should respond to them, value or avoid them. In the new 1948 British NHS, Norman Hartnell, the Queen's dress maker, designed hospital nurses' uniforms.[78] Previously, nun-like nurses' uniforms had echoed the long history of healthcare provided by religious and charitable institutions. Before Florence Nightingale began to reform non-religious nursing into a middle-class profession, many nurses were low-paid, low-status women, like the dirty drunken Sarah Gamp in Dickens's novel *Martin Chuzzlewit*. Nurses' currently continuing low pay enforces notions of nursing as a calling, a vocation of feminine caring, subordinate to the medical profession and still staffed mainly by women. Yet many nurses now have graduate degrees, while intensive nursing care, rather than surgical skill, mainly accounts for the present much higher postoperative survival rates. In their skill and knowledge, the closer parity of today's hospital nurses to doctors is shown by their unisex uniforms of 'scrubs'.

The changing cultural roles of nurses in their uniforms symbolise, reflect and reinforce how skilled, hygienic, scientific healthcare has increasingly come to be valued. Social attitudes of contempt or respect for nurses and their services shape and are shaped by related political and economic structures. Structure, agency and culture are all distinct, irreducible and in continuous interaction: structures and cultures constrain and enable agents' activity, and agents respond by conforming to the social order or by challenging or changing it.[79]

At the macro level, the power of cultural attitudes over economics and policies is shown by the 1984 Union Carbide tragedy in Bhopal, India.

> It remains the world's worst industrial disaster, which saw 40 tons of toxic methyl isocyanate gas released into the air, killing over 3,000 instantly and condemning hundreds of thousands to a future of prolonged pain, cancer, stillbirths, miscarriages, lung and heart disease and the drawn out deaths of everyone around them ... The official death toll is still disputed but an estimated 574,000 were poisoned that night and upwards of 20,000 people have died since from related conditions. No one from Union Carbide was ever tried for the gross negligence ... despite multiple criminal charges being brought against them. No cleanup operation of the chemical waste – which was being dumped into the local community well before the explosion – has ever been conducted.[80]

Lethal poisons continue to spread around the city, killing and disabling thousands more people even today. Decades of neglect can be attributed to attitudes and values. The Indian and US governments prevent and suppress research, assessments, and legal and practical action about Bhopal in order to protect the US company. They are supported by cultural global attitudes that value profits and Indian-US trade relations more than Indian individuals. The neo-colonial attitudes follow decades of richer countries outsourcing their low-paid industries, waste and pollution to poorer ones. Real change cannot occur solely at structural, or cultural, economic, legal, political or practical agential, levels. It has to be coordinated positively across all these levels, as powerfully as it is currently often coordinated and reinforced in negative ways.

Four types of social structures

Everyone acts from certain positions and relationships within four main constraining or enabling and motivating social structures identified by Douglas Porpora.[81]

1. Law-like regularities govern and determine social behaviours. Positivist and quantitative research and multivariate analysis follow Durkheim's view of structures as autonomous social facts, governed by their own laws and above agency. Actual behaviours and

events are measured. Covering law theory relies on consistently determining structures, such as Parsons's social system, Piaget's biological child development, Hume's constant conjunctions and Bourdieu's habitus.[82]

2. Structures as stable patterns involve innumerable activities and regular aggregate behaviours of agents over time. Structure is collapsed into agency or conflated with it in much interpretive research. This links to Margaret Thatcher's view that 'there is no such thing as society', only individuals and their repeated behaviours. This theory dominates economics, when assumedly selfish individuals sustain and regulate markets by their self-interest and pursuit of profit.
3. Structures are rules and resources, which individual agents draw on fairly freely, to structure or generate systematic patterns of relations and behaviours (structuration theory).[83] Archer criticises this reduction of structure into culture, which is the actual source of rules and resources. It also conflates structure with practices, so that structure, agency and culture all become one.[84] Porpora criticises this model, among other reasons, for neglecting research about how resources are distributed.[85] Culturally intersubjective schemas came to replace rules,[86] but Porpora considers schemas cannot replace objective material structures.
4. In CR theory, social structures are powerful, objective, enduring, material relations and resources among social positions and constructs that exist in and through human social relations. They far precede and outlast agents, who do not individually construct them but constantly reproduce or resist or modify them through their interactions with structures.[87]

Structures involve social positions that exist in relation to others; for example, social classes are defined in relation to one another:[88] those that own the means of production versus those that do not; the rentiers versus those who pay to use their amenities. Structural relations exist between those who plan, manage, fund, provide and sell health services and those who use them. Relations of competition or cooperation work within different supporting structures. Social structures connect to power struggles and relations that may be win-win (everyone gains) or zero-sum (the more one side gains, the more the other side loses, the usual economics model). Structures are understood in CR at the empirical, actual and especially the unseen real levels. These tend to be ignored in two main ways in positivist and interpretive research: in their concern with visible evidence in events or people's responses to them and in value-free or relativist ideologies that try to ignore the ethics and politics central to social structures and relations.

Theories of structure, agency and culture

CR theories about agency relate to daily experience. Our agency involves our enduring understanding and values and identity over time.[89] ANT and ethnomethodology 'bracket off' and disconnect examined events from the past. Yet if this really happened, readers would be unable to make sense of ANT reports. ANT researchers contradict and refute themselves when they have to rely on enduring, transferable, international reality-ontology, such as language or emails.

CR accepts that human agents are powerfully influenced by networks, powers, institutions, markets, cultures, assemblages and processes, that agency is sourced from multiple systems, things and other people, and that agency spreads out into its effects on others. Yet CR sites causal mechanisms of agency within as well as between agents. Do we have rights and any control over our agency or must we rely on others to mediate, construct and interpret it? To answer these questions, a little of Archer's CR work on agency will be summarised.

Social structure, agency and culture (SAC) can only exist in relation to each other.[90] They are separate and distinct but interacting, partly overlapping but irreducible. Without values and resources from structures and culture to enable us to make sense of experience, agency would be empty or chaotic, meaningless and overwhelming. Agents live in competing structures in open systems where independent intransitive structures interact with agents' transitive responses.

Archer warns against conflation,[91] the confusing and blurring together of things that are actually separate. Unless they are seen to be distinct, their interactions cannot be understood, because after things merge or are conflated together they no longer interact. For example, salt and water can change each another, but once they become salty water that interaction ceases. Salt loses its dry strong-tasting properties and water its neutral tastelessness. If agents and structures are conflated, agents lose their conscious intentions while inanimate structures are invested with fake powers. There are three kinds of structure-agency conflation.

1. In downward conflation, or structural determinism, structures dominate over the people who are merged into the structures. This is the positivist tradition of Durkheim, Parsons and Bourdieu's *habitus*, quantitative mass surveys, and statistical analysis.

Determining if not determinist social structures are assumed to shape human life and society. Researchers attend to conditions rather than actions.

2. In upward conflation or voluntarism, people freely orchestrate the structures. Researchers attend to actions but not enough to conditions-structures, which are merged into the agents. In Weber's interpretive tradition, agents shape human life and society, and structures are the resources they freely draw on.
3. In central conflation, Giddens's structuration theory, structure and agents are merged and mutually constituted so that their interactions cannot be adequately understood and researched.

CR recognises how structure, culture and agency are separate, distinct and interacting, not merged or conflated. This vital distinction was shown in the English film *I, Daniel Blake*.[92] Daniel's doctor told him he was too ill to work and must rest, whereas the universal credit (or unemployment benefit) staff told him he must apply for work while they denied him benefits. The film follows Daniel's many attempts to care for himself until he died. The impact of powerful social structures – the universal credit system where computer programmes control claimants and staff, the government austerity policies, the shrinking of the welfare state and social housing, and the fragmenting of communities – are central to understanding the causes of Daniel's death. They show how clear analysis depends on avoiding conflation of social structure and agency as if they are interchangeable, discussed in the next section.

Realist evaluation, critical realism, structure and agency

RE and CR approaches will be compared because, as mentioned earlier, RE is widely used in health research and illustrates differences and similarities between CR and other paradigms.[93] The CMO (context-mechanism-outcome) theory in RE conflates structure and agency, resources and reasoning,[94] whereas Bhaskar distinguishes

> between the genesis of human actions, lying in the reasons, intentions and plans of human beings, on the one hand; and the structures governing the reproduction and transformation of social activities, on the other.[95]

Noting this, the critical realist Samuel Porter questioned Pawson's concept of programme mechanisms.[96] These merge together 'pre-existing structure [with] the limited, emerging relations that can follow under human interpretation'.[97] Porter considers that differences between CR and RE 'are not as significant as Pawson contends'. The main differences concern social structures-human agency and facts-values.[98]

Porter noted that CR sites social causal mechanisms 'exclusively within the structural component of the social world' separate from agency.[99] However, RE social mechanisms combine agency with structure and 'are thus about people's choices and the capacities they derive from group membership'.[100] Porter added:

> Agents, while they both influence and are influenced by these social systems, are different, not least because they have the capacity to think and choose while social structures do not ... While social mechanisms will undoubtedly impinge upon people's choices, they are not the mechanisms involved in the making of choices, which reside in the psyches of individuals.[101]

Porter agrees that, as discussed in Chapter 1, research programme mechanisms constructed in Pawson's RE cannot be either agents or (structural) causal mechanisms because 'they have been consciously created by agents', the researchers. Porter disagrees with the RE claim that its programmes entail 'the interplay between social resources and participants' reasoning' because these have been conflated in RE.[102] Yet 'participants' reasoning ... is categorically distinct' from their resources,[103] and CR's structure-agency dualism 'rescues agency' from the CMO formula and 'confusion', when CMO conflates

> agency and structure under the rubric of 'mechanism' [which] means that it cannot sufficiently recognize the capacity of humans to choose, and is thus an inadequate description of causal chains in the social world ... I propose that agency should be included as a separate category alongside context and mechanism in the [CMO] evaluation formula.[104]

Structure-agency dialectic

In CR, structure-agency interaction or dialectic shapes human life and society. A comparison is a river flowing through a landscape, like individuals flowing through their society in their lifetime. Does the river shape the land around it or does the land shape the river?

Do individuals shape their social contexts or are they shaped by them? Structures, such as hospitals, precede the agents who use them and work in them and outlast the agents. But they can only exist as hospitals, not empty buildings, through the activities of the agents who reproduce, resist or modify them. Structures are determining (very powerful) but not determinist (final arbiters or sole causes), because they compete in open systems of many different forces.

CR analysis is neither voluntarist (over-free agency) nor determinist (over-passive agency); it is interactive through structure-agency dialectic. With our limited agency, we live in conditions not of our own choosing,[105] and we are 'thrown' into our social contexts. Thrownness is Heidegger's concept of how we enter pre-existing, often alienating, fast-moving social life, and it tended to emphasise structures over agency, past over present. CR extends Heidegger's thrownness also to emphasise agency, ethics and the dynamic pulse of freedom.[106] Yet our actions often have unintended, counterproductive, unwanted and unpredicted effects.[107]

A vital CR insight is that agents' motives and reasons can be powerful causal mechanisms. This transforms humans from being the puppets of structures and variables into being motivated influential agents. Agency means to act, do, set in motion and cause intentionally. However strong the external influences on their health, individuals' choices about when, how, why and what they eat also affect their health. Agency's causal power is informed by human intention and purpose, orientated to and evaluated by future effects.[108] To cause is also to absent, to remove certain things or states in order to introduce new ones; becomings involve begoings.[109] To become healthy involves overcoming or absenting ill-health; vaccinations absent the risk of infections; chemotherapy absents cancer. They involve working from power2 towards power1 and also towards theory-practice consistency in harmony with personal values. However, agents' interests may differ and conflict so that actions that serve one group may harm others.

Agency's two main concerns occur over time. First, causal intention precedes action, which, second, is often followed by reflexive monitoring of the intended and actual effects, the basis for future action.[110] Positivist and interpretive concepts of agency are often fixed and static, whereas CR shows how agency works and changes over time. Like the river-landscape interaction, agents and structures are shaped and reshaped through dialectical processes.

One CR model is Bhaskar's TMSA, the transformational model of social activity (Figure 3.1). Individuals move or are thrown into social contexts through which they are socialised, and they then react by

Figure 3.1: Transformational model of social activity

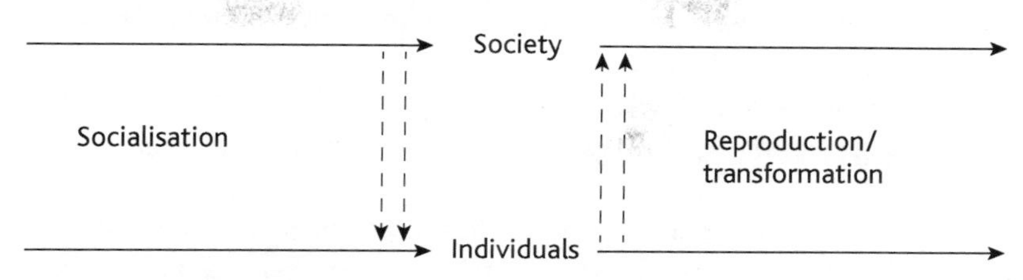

Source: Bhaskar, 1998 [1979]: 36

reproducing or transforming society. The process occurs in countless, continuous, multiple cycles.

Another version is Archer's morphostasis and morphogenesis,[111] from morph (form, structure), stasis (static, present state) and genesis (origins, birth, change). Agents conform to and reinforce (stasis) or resist, change and reconstruct (genesis) structures. Like TMSA, the morphogenetic cycle involves structural conditioning leading to social interaction leading to structural elaboration. Objective structures pre-exist agents and provide resources, interests, roles and values. Agents cause effects through their personal emergent properties. Unlike structures and objects, agents are self-aware, reflexive and intentional. They are objectively real, but subjective by nature.

The three levels of natural necessity help with analysing the three levels of agency and of agency-structure interaction (Table 3.1).

Table 3.1: Agency, structure and natural necessity

	Agency	Agency↔Structure
Empirical	Experiences of agency Embodied impressions, sensations, images, evaluations, memories, making meaning of sensed experience	Experiences of social and natural structures that enable and constrain agency Inner conversations (see below)
Actual	Activity, making choices and decisions, chains of events, interactions, relationships	Agency-structure interactions Actual social structures existing through agency
Real causal mechanisms	Agency shaped by genes and environment, personal needs, relationships, reasons and motives	Natural, social, political, economic cultures and structures; causes of illness and disability

Example 3.1 illustrates the morphogenetic cycle in research with prison leavers.

Example 3.1 Using the morphogenetic cycle to evaluate a complex intervention for prison leavers with common mental health problems

Sarah Rybczynska-Bunt, Lauren Weston and Richard Byng
Community and Primary Care Research Group, University of Plymouth, UK[112]

Engager is a complex health intervention. It is used to support the wellbeing of offenders who have common mental health problems, near to and after their release from prison. Our evaluation of a trial of Engager used the morphogenetic cycle to research prison leavers' initial responses to the intervention, when, where and how it might begin to take effect, and interactions with social contexts.[113] Can Engager be flexible and can it offer person-centred support?

During the Engager trial in 2016–17 there were significant cutbacks to council budgets and criminal justice services. Consequently there was very little support for prison leavers after short-term sentences. Engager was meant to fill a gap in service provision when there was less integrated working with other services.

Engager practitioners had experience in different social services, and they had basic MBA (Mentalisation-Based Approach) training and supervision, though they often had limited therapeutic experience.

We examined four themes.

- **Engagement and trust**: practitioners offered a range of practical and emotional supports to build trust.
- **Meeting at the gate**: practitioners supported participants on the day they left prison to help them procure resources and engage with relevant community services.
- **The shared understanding:** practitioners helped participants develop an understanding of how their thoughts, emotions and impulses drive behaviour, informing a shared understanding of the participant's current strengths, resources, difficulties and things to work on.
- **The shared action** plan relates to using resources to support the personal goals.

The trial participants in our evaluation had or were at acute risk of having common mental health problems. However, they varied widely in the number of stressors they had to cope with. Some had the support of families and friends, housing and perhaps job prospects to return to, while others had little support and were at acute risk of homelessness, relapse and reoffending. They all served short sentences, two years or less; many had previous convictions. We evaluated two sites, one urban and one semi-rural. We tested the Engager logic model through 24 case studies. We conducted qualitative and quantitative interviews with participants at multiple time points, with their family-friends, Engager practitioners and other service practitioners working with the individual.

We began with antecedent events: the social contexts, the stressors and participant's initial response to intervention offers. At stage two, we explored 'temporal interactions', which involves examining the initial responses to offers of support from Engager practitioners.

Some participants reported having no support on past prison releases and they were keen to see whether this might help them abstain from substance misuse in the community. Others were uncertain that they would maintain engagement with their practitioner. They often seemed to be resigned to accepting that their lives were unlikely to improve. They lacked self-efficacy and felt unable to make positive changes.

Participants with some social capital often thought they did not need Engager support after they left prison. Practitioners appeared to struggle to challenge some of the participants' thinking, or else they believed that the prison leavers were relatively self-reflexive about the challenges facing them. Despite best-laid plans, these participants often could not sustain change as the pressures on them mounted.

Building trust with participants needed time, not simply in the sheer amount of contacts offered but in practitioners competently gauging the participant's upmost concerns and responding appropriately at that moment in time. Motivation often ebbed and practitioners needed to respond to fluctuating moods. They gave consistent support and their MBA skills were sometimes useful in helping participants to reflect on their feelings, thinking and behaviours, which often helped to renew their motivation to continue to pursue their goals. Other practitioners felt disheartened by the participant's low mood, and lack of a strong underlying motivation they believed was needed in order to make best use of the support offered. A failure to appeal to participants in these initial interactions thus often maintained a morphostasis.

Stage three, 'directional interaction', was the beginning of the intervention effects. Practitioners often had to tread a fine balance between 'acceptance' and 'change', by being inquisitive about a person's experiences, thoughts and feelings, without judgement or assumption, while gently pushing for change through establishing goals and exploring obstacles and solutions.[114] However, they and the trial design may have underestimated the time needed to achieve behavioural changes. Lack of progress sometimes left practitioners feeling discouraged, which often adversely affected their work. Morphostasis could turn into negative morphogenesis, which unintentionally reinforced participants' despair.

Time is also important when practitioners must gauge when to offer resources. For example, one participant soon after leaving prison appeared to make little progress and arrived at sessions intoxicated. If his practitioner had pushed for change when his self-efficacy was low, he would have most likely decided that he could not make or sustain the changes. However, the practitioner listened and empathised to the challenges rather than trying to 'fix' or 'change' his behaviour that same day. This enabled the participant to reflect on his difficulties and he started bridging connections between maladaptive coping strategies and his thoughts and feelings. He identified that he drank more on days leading up to an appointment, to manage his anxiety. This understanding enabled him to develop coping strategies to manage appointments and over time significantly lowered his alcohol intake.

At stage four, Archer contends that while relatively enduring structures cannot be eradicated they can be reshaped and elaborated through morphogenesis. Interventions such as Engager might alter systems of support for prison leavers, though one time-limited trial would have little effect on criminal justice services generally. Nevertheless, some practitioners from other services changed how they worked with individuals. For instance, by accompanying a participant to key appointments, Engager practitioners helped to model more positive communication. Their sustained and positive engagement with offender managers often led to less restrictions and more flexibility.

While practitioners from other services did not explicitly report that they had changed their working practices, some did acknowledge a marked change in the way the participant positively engaged with the service compared with previous experience. Therefore, Engager may have demonstrated that a new way of working, based on a shared understanding, may provide some individuals with psychological competencies to: identify and articulate their thoughts, feelings and needs; interrelate better with services; pursue their goals and potentially desist from crime through positive morphogenesis.

Internal conversations

Valuable non-CR research has shown the importance of inner reflections and retelling of personal stories. Peter Fonagy helped individuals with brittle Type I diabetes to improve their self-healthcare. He believed they mismanaged their daily care because they did not have any other language than self-harm through which to express their difficulties and distress. By deeply understanding their view of the world he helped them, individually and in groups, to find emotional control and a positive reflective language of mentalisation, which he considers works in all effective psychological and psychoanalytical methods.[115] Another internal conversation is qualitative researchers' reflexive processes that CR can help to extend.

Enduring individual agency exists over time in several ways. It is emergent. The brain has emerged from the body, the mind from the physical brain and consciousness from mind. Each level is interdependent and irreducible.[116] Each higher order is more complex than lower ones and cannot be explained by them. Our consciousness is partly informed by our bodies but not wholly explained by them.

Bhaskar saw agency, each 'moment in a person's life', in tiers: biology; the unconscious, preconscious and self-conscious; up through more layers of reflexivity and praxis; up to society, nature, the biosphere and the cosmos.[117] SEPM, synchronic emergent powers materialism, resolves mind/body abstract/physical dichotomies into mind-body dialectic. The mind emerges from the brain in synchronicity (concurrently).[118] Neuroscience might one day solve the mystery of consciousness, but meanwhile CR philosophy avoids either solely physical or abstract terms. It stresses the process when beliefs and desires inform an individual's choices and behaviour through consciousness, showing that reasons can be causes. CR thereby avoids the false choices often posed by multidisciplinary research between 'causation and freedom, reductive materialism and defensive idealism'.[119] (Chapter 6 considers emergence and interdisciplinary research.)

Archer identified a major structure-agency interaction: agents draw on structures for knowledge and choices, inwardly consider them and then make personal decisions about outward action. Serious decisions are not made on a casual pick-and-mix basis. They invoke what really matters to that person, drawing on lasting personal values.[120] An example is when people choose consistently to buy vegetarian food or when they choose to give up unhealthy food. The choices can be costly, not just in price but in time and in relationships. They may involve no longer eating with friends or family but finding new like-minded friends when sharing meals.

The decisions and choices are not only about what to do, or what to have, but more seriously they are about ontology: 'What kind of person do I want to be?'[121] This involves identifying oneself, and being willing to be identified, as a vegetarian. The transition from unhealthy to healthy lifestyles involves complex personal and social changes of identity. This partly explains why people may find support from course leaders or peers more helpful than an actual course on health living.[122] CR analysis supports healthcare professionals who do not simply prescribe and instruct about healthy living but who also listen and negotiate. Their patients' choices may be misinformed but are nevertheless based on personal logic and values that need to be discussed and reconsidered.

Archer traced internal structure-agency interactions through her interviewees' accounts of their continual inner conversations.[123] These involve how 'our personal emergent powers are exercised on and in the world—natural, practical and social—which is our triune environment'.[124] We each have unique individuality in our concrete (actual) singularity.[125] Archer identified how we all individually draw and reflect on objective structures through four types of subjective conversations when we make conclusions or decisions.

1. Autonomous reflexivity: people are independent and decide on their actions with little discussion.
2. Communicative reflexivity: they consult and discuss with others.
3. Meta-reflexivity: they are highly thoughtful and self-aware of their extended thinking.
4. Fractured reflexivity: people cannot resolve uncertainties and dilemmas. Their reflexivity is impeded or displaced, lost in fraught emotions or passive helplessness.

The internal conversations illustrate how CR analysis of structure-agency dialectic avoids problems in some other paradigms. Unlike them, CR examines:

- real agents, distinct from determining (but not determinist) structures, showing the central role of agency in human activity;
- lifelong identities that change only partly and with difficulty, never wholly, unlike some hermeneutic theories that assume identities are constantly reconstructed;[126]
- intensely active, aware, personal agency, unlike postmodern theories of absent, unaware, dispersed or multiple agency;[127]
- agents who apply language and are influenced but not constructed by language or by Foucauldian discourse or micro-technologies (the surveillance of the prison or the confessional);

- agents' complex reflections and reasons that precede their activities, unlike ANT reduction of human agents to the level of inanimate objects; and
- agency-structure dialectic that avoids voluntarism (strong agents and weak structures) or determinism (over-strong structures and weak agents).

Archer's theories can be adapted to many kinds of health and illness research. Example 3.2 explores nurses' documentation in relation to morphogenesis.

Example 3.2: Exploring nurses' documentation of their contribution to traumatic brain injury rehabilitation

Angela Davenport, Auckland University of Technology, New Zealand[128]

I used a critical realist organisational case study framework.[129] During data analysis, I applied Archer's (1995) morphogenetic analytical framework. I drew on international research about nurses' contribution in the rehabilitation setting.[130] However, there was little research about what daily work rehabilitation nurses actually document and why they choose to document it in the way they do. Archer's framework highlighted the complexity in nurses' decision-making relating to this component of their daily practice. It enabled analysis beyond the identification of documentation themes to consider contextual and causal factors and influences.

Many rehabilitation facilities audit documentation practice to ensure clarity and completeness. Initially, I had considered comparing actual practice against documentation patterns or analysing documentation data from multiple facilities. However, this would not describe the contextual and causal factors and influences. At the time of my research, New Zealand funding criteria separated nursing care from nurses' rehabilitative input, and this distinction was also not always made in the literature.[131]

I used a single case embedded design for in-depth analysis of one rehabilitation facility.[132] I gained ethics approval. The facility name was kept confidential and I only had access to anonymised data. The research was undertaken in three phases. Phase A: an environmental description of the facility, including the funding contract, local policy documents and a questionnaire for two managers. Phase B: analysis of nurses' documentation in the electronic client record. Phase C: six nurses were interviewed about their view of their role and the documentation choices they made. They also gave their perspective of the differences in the way they worked with the data from Phases A and B. I also asked about their expectations as well as the enablers and constraints of their documentation practice.

Nurses' written records demonstrated an impersonal style of documentation, where their interactions with the client were not evident. Additionally, the nurses tended to prioritise documenting information that they believed was legally important. However, this style of documentation provided little basis for readers to recognise how nurses were uniquely involved in a client's rehabilitation progress.[133] For example, rather than detailing how rehabilitative input was provided and the client's responses to what was done, it was written '*Care given as per protocol. Sat in chair for most of the morning. Pain meds given prior to physio. Incontinence needs met.*' The way nurses documented their practices contrasted with how they talked about their strong sense of value in their work with their clients. One nurse commented, '*I don't do paperwork very well! And I don't like that to disrupt or take away anything that I'm doing with my clients,*'[134] showing how they prioritised their clinical practice role over documentation requirements.

Following initial data analysis of the three phases, I applied Archer's morphogenetic analytical framework to understand causal mechanisms that were influencing the nurses' documentation practice.[135] Separating structure, culture and agency and Archer's notion of primary and corporate agency increased my awareness of nurses' individual and shared understandings and responses. The nurses articulated different understandings of their rehabilitative role and individually interpreted facility requirements relating to their documentation. Individually and collectively, nurses could have transformed their documentation practice, but structures, cultures, and social interactions inhibited this and morphostasis of existing documentation practices continued.

Summary

Structure or agency, positivism or interpretivism, quantity or quality, all tend to be separated or imbalanced in misleading, one-sided research reports. CR shows how more realistic and useful research examines the complementary interactions of all these dyads in larger contexts. Social disadvantages can be seen as tendencies and processes, and powerful latent forces, but they do not always predominate and may often be overridden by other social forces in open systems. It is therefore vital to research complex structure-agency interactions. Quantitative measures of poverty levels need to be combined with qualitative research about their detailed effects. Much non-CR research combines these dyads. Mentalisation research, for example, involves case studies and RCTs, individuals and broader views of the world.[136]

CR helps to explain and resolve underlying contradictions between the research paradigms and to extend their work on individual, social and physical understandings of human agency (in this chapter), of agency across space (Chapter 5), across time (Chapter 6) and in potential future alternatives (Chapter 7). The next chapter considers morality in agency and society.

Questions to write or talk about with colleagues

1. Divide a page into three parts. How do your main concerns about agency, culture and structure in your research fit into each part?
2. How does your own experience confirm or deny the different theories of agency and of structure?
3. Which model of agency and of structure do you prefer?
4. How does your research look at agents and structures? Which seem to be more powerful?
5. How could the six features of CR inform your research?
6. How could analysis of the four kinds of reflexivity or four kinds of social structures inform your research?

4

Health and illness research: value-free or value-laden?

> Child poverty is a key indicator of ill health throughout life. A report about hungry families in Britain recounted young people's shame, guilt and sense of exclusion from normal, everyday activities. Bryony, aged 13, living with her mother and brother said about meal times, 'It gets a bit to the point where we'll start feeling guilty because Mum hasn't had anything and we've had it'.[1]

The poverty researchers assumed that accurate reports about hunger include people's moral responses. Mary O'Hara contends that powerful groups maintain inequalities partly by the moral blaming and shaming of the poor.[2] The rich claim ceaselessly that they are the brightest and best and the hardest working group. They deserve their wealth and can be trusted to manage it, unlike the feckless poor.

> Shame is how they get away with it. Shame is the weapon they use. Shame is the weapon you use on yourself that makes you feel so useless. And those who are shamed most often and most deeply, made to feel ashamed for so much of their life, are the poorest among us.[3]

Just before the 2020 pandemic:

> In the UK, numbers of working families in poverty are at an all time high. They rely on benefits from a state system that is driving many more of them into debt and to use food banks, and some to starvation and suicide.[4]

This chapter is about how critical realism (CR) addresses values in health research and helps to extend moral analyses. Health research that describes, measures and provides much vital information is necessary but not sufficient. Research is also needed to explain driving moral forces and how adverse forces might be changed.

This chapter considers: if facts can be separated from values; health-related rights; dignity; truth, trust and consent; values and then ethics in health research and what CR can add; health research paradigms and ethics; ethical naturalism and moral realism; learning from other major theorists: advocacy on many levels and, finally, realist evaluation (RE), CR and values. First, value-freedom is considered.

Can and should research be value-free?

Typically, a British Parliamentary report *The Health of the Nation* assumed a moral consensus:[5] that premature death should be prevented and longevity promoted equally among all social groups. The report cited economic and social benefits and advised that 'reducing this gap [in unequal health and survival rates] would therefore generate substantial gross value-added, estimated at an additional £13.2bn' when the productivity of healthier workers would improve, besides other social advantages. Disputes arise about the methods of achieving these benefits.

All health research is value-laden in its implicit direct or indirect aim: to reduce and prevent suffering by promoting health and wellbeing. Much interdisciplinary natural science research similarly aims to promote and conserve the health of the fragile ecosphere and of most species.[6] Yet the idea that research can and should be value-free is widespread.

Here are eight approaches to values by social scientists.

1. Just as positivism and interpretivism conceal being within thinking (ontology within epistemology), they also conceal values within facts. Objectivity is taken to mean value-free. Yet 'objective' can mean impartial, fair, open-minded, rigorously enquiring and setting aside personal interests as much as possible but need not mean being value-free. Indeed all those standards, along with honesty and accuracy, are values that scientists prize.
2. Many researchers believe facts can be tested through reasoned analysis, but values are too vague and subjective to be rational.
3. Behaviourism involves observing objects, events and behaviours but not human meanings, motives or values. Someone can be described as 'kneeling' but not as 'praying', 'honouring' or 'begging for help'. Behaviourist research that sets aside intentions can deny real human agency and become 'self-blinding'.[7] An honoured psychologist found her research on persuading individuals consciously to reduce their risky behaviours produced 'null findings'. She switched

to researching risk information that 'targeted non-conscious [irrational] as opposed to the conscious processes' and promoted 'nudge' government policies.[8] This raises ethical questions about disrespect for participants' informed consent and human agency.

4. Beehive-like functionalism assumes that everything functions for the common good in smoothly run societies.[9] Research may show how to make processes more efficient and cost-effective but not how to question or change oppressive ones. Insistence on visible 'evidence-base' can exclude unseen values and better missing alternatives. When 'deviants' include patients who should get well and be re-socialised into productive work,[10] they are not seen as potentially useful critics of failing systems. Functionalists assume it is correctly neutral to avoid questioning dominant power and policies but ignore how they thereby inevitably support the policies.
5. Functionalists are utilitarian when they value each part according to its function or utility. Values and power are then not excluded but may covertly be connected to wealth, control and cost-effectiveness rather than to wisdom, justice and compassion.[11] Utilitarians concentrate on outcomes when the ends can justify harsh means. Researchers may not question austerity programmes designed to reduce future national debts, although austerity can greatly increase mortality and morbidity rates.
6. Social constructionists and ethnographers aim for understanding, *Verstehen*,[12] of anyone's viewpoint without judgement.[13] This can also risk seeming to endorse unjust or coercive practices.
7. When social constructionists believe that all values are socially constructed and emerge from and make sense only within local contexts, they accept moral relativism.[14] In this view, nothing is real, or if there is any reality it can only be contingent and make sense in a specific context, not elsewhere. Yet as noted in Chapter 3, this claim is self-defeating when relativist researchers publish reports in international journals. It is dangerous to deny universal meanings, values and rights on which researchers rely in their private life to defend against plagiarism, or theft, or invasion of privacy.

Moral relativism, which denies any universal rights and values, is sometimes termed 'cultural relativism'. Yet cultural relativism does respect universal values and can judge each culture by universal standards. However, it does not take its own culture as the sole standard and willingly criticises it if another culture seems more humane. The anthropologist Margaret Mead criticised stressful conditions for young people in her own US and admired the relaxed carefree life that Samoan young people enjoyed.[15]

Respectful cultural relativism assists the study of unhealthy group behaviours. Instead of simply telling communities to avoid dead bodies during Ebola epidemics to reduce cross-infection, interpretivists study how and why people observe religious and cultural customs when caring for the deceased. They show how these customs are highly valued, with the need to negotiate respectfully with local people about changing the customs, if cross-infection is to be reduced.[16] Sada Mire's archaeological (also non-CR) study in North-East Africa revealed relations between 'sacred fertility', FGM (female genital mutilation), spirit possessions and other physically invasive rituals.[17] These enabled Mire to suggest ways to replace harmful traditions with new rituals.

8. Critical theory and CR accept that, unlike the beehive harmony of functionalism, societies are riven with inequalities and injustice and often conflicting ideas about justice. Everyone competes at times for scarce resources, power or control.[18] Human relations are not all benign. Respect for universal values and rights is essential when arbitrating claims and disputes to promote freedom and justice.[19]

These eight approaches indicate how morality runs through social research, whether researchers acknowledge it or not. To suppose moral neutrality ignores but cannot delete values, and risks by default reinforcing present powerful structures and inequalities.

Can facts be separated from values?

Facts are often taken to be real things, whereas they are statements, truth claims that may or may not be accurate. To assume that facts exist independently involves the epistemic fallacy, which confuses the idea with the reality it describes. Facts depend on the value of truth that is honestly believed. When critics, fallibilists or sceptics test facts for their veracity, in effect, they all measure the fact by how near to or far from some independent truth it may be.

Hyper-factual positivists and hypo-factual interpretivists were contrasted earlier. They both try to separate 'objective facts' from 'subjective values'. Interpretivists limit the certainty and relevance of ideas to certain contexts. Positivists follow Hume's edict that science must be value-free: you cannot derive an 'is' from an 'ought', and there is no coherent move from a description to any prescription based on normative values.[20] Yet Hume's edict does what he forbids, when he writes 'I shall presume to recommend' what his readers ought and ought not to do. To derive 'is' from 'ought' is a common practice, so it is not impossible, just prohibited in the 'ought not' sense. Hume believed facts and values must be separate because '[I] am persuaded, that this small attention would subvert all the vulgar systems of morality, and let us see, that the distinction of vice and virtue is not founded merely on the relations of objects, nor is perceived by reason'.[21] So Hume asserted that unseen morality is neither empirical nor rational.[22] Yet subjective health scientists select or develop facts through making practical and moral choices about their relevance, aiming to avoid deceit and plagiarism and hoping their work will be believed, respected and might have positive influence.

Many philosophers reject Hume's edict.[23] CR shares their criticisms by showing how attempts to distance facts from values raise theory-practice inconsistencies and problems of double standards.[24] Moral values do not prevent wrong-doing, but they define them as wrong and support the means of preventing them. Societies depend on these values, and what value can research have if it tries to ignore them? Theory-practice consistency is essential for communication, discovery, autonomy, flourishing and social progress. Bhaskar equates it with justice because it expresses our real moral selves and avoids hypocrisy, although he approves of Nietzsche's honest admission: 'From the beginning we are unlogical and therefore unjust beings and we can know this: this is one of the greatest and most insoluble disharmonies of existence.'[25] There is constant dialectic between failure, self-awareness and hope.

How do values matter?

Each year seemingly neutral facts and choices that underlie trade, transport, fashion and many other aspects of daily life become more obviously morally loaded. The adverse impact of food industries includes exploited workers, pollution, global heating and harm to the health of and survival of humans and many other species.[26] The critical realist Andrew Sayer sees how social life is imbued with morality because we are evaluative beings concerned with health and flourishing and suffering. The attempt to separate facts from values in supposedly moral neutrality is folly.[27]

> Imagine going to the doctor to have your blood pressure taken. She does so and gives you two numbers, one over

> the other. You say, 'Is that good or bad? What should I do about it?' Imagine if the doctor answered, 'Well, I can't tell you because that would be a value judgment and it would compromise my objectivity, and I can't advise you what to do because you can't derive an ought from an is.'[28]

We can never fully know or suspend all our values. Many are held subconsciously. Some may be central to the research, such as when investigating dangerous or corrupt health services. It is vital to be as critically aware of our values as possible, to acknowledge them, test them against the evidence and be willing to change them if necessary.

The ethnographer Martyn Hammersley contends that researchers should not make moral judgements, such as to assume that starving people who (factually) might die therefore (morally) ought to be fed. He asks, 'What if they are an oppressive army?',[29] a moral question. He adds that researchers 'should strive to be value neutral or objective' in their own work while accepting 'that value argument … is essential to governance and to everyday life'. Yet Hammersley does not explain his own value judgement that researchers 'ought' to avoid the complex moral questions inherent in everyday social research. It is not a matter of introducing values into the data but of recognising the integral values already present. To avoid them would collapse the intransitive ontology of real values, as causes of human interactions, into the transitive epistemology, as if values are simply expendable ideas, not realities.

Andrew Sayer questions why researchers are supposed to suspend their humanity when at work.[30] He notes the double standards (theory-practice contradictions) mentioned earlier, which risk breaking the golden rule of always treating others (including participants, readers and potential beneficiaries of the research) with the same justice and respect as you would expect to be treated yourself.[31] Even 'objective' research involves the values of veracity and accuracy, of being fair and impartial when openly listening with mutual trust and respect, trying to understand and report every side. But that need not mean valuing everything neutrally, evenly and inconclusively, or overlooking cruelty and injustice, or remaining silent about them. 'A politics without ethics can embrace genocide as easily as democracy.'[32]

Detached scientists can only distort or close understanding if they refuse to value nature's beauty and integrity; destructive applied science and technology show the dangers of this denial. Health researchers who value their subject matter can become more deeply aware of it. A cancer researcher wrote of becoming absorbed in her subject, as if she was touching 'something central' to it. 'One feels silent and grateful ... because one was allowed to penetrate a layer of understanding which remained impenetrable to others ... If you really want to understand about a tumour, you've got to *be* a tumour.'[33] Another researcher wrote that organisms do everything we can think of 'better, more efficiently, more marvellously'.[34] And that may apply still more to human individuals and groups.

Another questionable normative part of health research involves whose interests are served in the selection of research questions and granting of funds. Pharmaceutical companies over-fund substandard research designed to 'prove' their products are effective and refuse to publish reports of ineffective treatments. They spend billions of dollars on researching drugs to ease Western lifestyles that already suffer from controversial over-prescriptions.[35] They neglect to develop vaccines and treatments greatly needed by billions of people in low-income countries.[36] 'Me-too' research tweaks the ingredients of medications so that 'new' versions of drugs can be 'discovered' and lucrative patents can be renewed. This prevents the drugs from being sold far more cheaply once the patents have expired.[37] Universities' R&D and ethics review systems support this commerce that exploits research likely to increase their income and prestige.[38]

The fact/value split leads many positivists to evade moral questions about power and interests that relate political economies to rising morbidity rates.[39] For decades, scientists such as Michael Marmot on health inequalities and David Attenborough on the climate crisis spoke as if their often shocking evidence could and should speak for itself and persuade their viewers and readers to take their findings seriously enough to make personal and political changes.[40] But concerned about the lack of change, they recently began to speak more politically. This can be difficult for leading scientists. They want to keep the confidence of the public, the government, their peers, sponsors and funders by being 'proper' and therefore value-free apolitical scientists who stay within their narrow area of expertise. Positivists' mistaken attempts to split facts from values can lead to their bolting on ethical and political analysis as a later extra, whereas for CR researchers these are integral throughout the research. Marmot recently challenged the positivist tradition and urged the government to put wellbeing, not fiscal growth, at the heart of policy.[41] He said:

> We have to make sure that we change the agenda, we take the action, that we *don't* sit back and say 'how will it come out?' We convince politicians, the policy makers, as well as

> our communities, that we are serving in the cause of social justice and health equity. And what greater cause could there be than that?[42]

If researchers are unaware of their values, these can unduly influence the research. This was shown by a (non-CR) evaluation of public engagement exercises for the government,[43] which found:

1. the market researchers who consulted the public selected their focus groups guided by beliefs about 'a strongly imagined public as neither overly critical nor supportive';
2. the researchers' overt aims, 'such as including publics in developing ethical data regulations, were overshadowed by' covert aims, 'such as counteracting public fears';
3. all concerned 'understood the term "engagement" in varying ways, from creating interest to public inclusion';
4. government hopes for a positive report, influenced what was written in the final report, which sought to 'benefit government and technical stakeholders rather than publics'; and
5. public engagement exercises can 'shut down opportunities for meaningful public dialogue'.

Concern for equality goes beyond equal treatment regardless of need and beyond equity when treatment differs according to need. Equality as justice involves removing the structures that create inequalities.[44] Official bodies are making more moral and political statements about equality. The Royal College of Physicians has 'urgently' called on the government to take Marmot's 'shocking' findings seriously and to increase the minimum wage and end child poverty.[45] CR analysis of the power and values integral to healthcare helps to validate these moves, which involve respecting human rights.

Health-related rights

There is no 'right to health'. It is an empty slogan (like the 'right to love'), which critics may deride to discredit rights. CR is useful in promoting clearer analysis of human rights, through the empirical, actual and real levels. Empirically, human rights are legal concepts, framed in ways that can be defended in courts of law. It would be pointless to say to someone dying of cancer, 'don't worry, you have a right to health', because health (and love) cannot be willed or enforced. The more realistic wording is everyone's right 'to the enjoyment of the highest attainable standard of physical and mental health'.[46] This can involve terminally ill people being kept as comfortable as possible.

Rights entail governments respecting and protecting everyone's,[47] or at least their citizens', rights.[48] The *Universal Declaration of Human Rights (UDHR)* states:

> Everyone has the right to a standard of living adequate for the health and wellbeing of himself [*sic*] and of his family, including food, clothing, housing and medical care and necessary social services, and the right to security in the event of unemployment, sickness, disability, widowhood, old age or other lack of livelihood in circumstances beyond his control.[49]

Like its partner report, the 1947 *Nuremberg Code* on ethical standards for medical research, the *UDHR* set a global programme of decades of work to promote and assure human rights.[50] In 1989, the *UN Convention on the Rights of the Child (UNCRC)* spelt out children's rights at empirical and actual levels.

> States Parties shall ... take appropriate measures:
> (a) To diminish infant and child mortality;
> (b) To ensure the provision of necessary medical assistance and health care to all children with emphasis on the development of primary health care;
> (c) To combat disease and malnutrition, including within the framework of primary health care ... the application of readily available technology and through the provision of adequate nutritious foods and clean drinking-water, taking into consideration the dangers and risks of environmental pollution ...[51]

High-income countries are called on to assist low-income ones, which would reverse the trend of healthcare professionals expensively trained in low-income countries moving to high-income ones. Babies do not have the right to breastfeed, which could violate their mothers' embodied rights. Instead they have the right that everyone,

> in particular parents and children, are informed, have access to education and are supported in the use of basic knowledge of child health and nutrition, the advantages of breastfeeding, hygiene and environmental sanitation and the prevention of accidents ...[52]

CR analysis of rights at the actual level recognises the ontology, or the being and doing, of human rights. Most rights are embodied. They concern feeding, clothing and housing bodies, treating sick and disabled bodies, defending them from unjust constraints, from humiliating and degrading treatment, from torture and wrongful imprisonment. Even seemingly abstract rights, such as freedom of information and expression and the right to make peaceful protest, depend on bodies. They are enabled to access information through the five senses, attend school and express protest through writing, talking, singing and street demonstrations. Eleanor Roosevelt, an early promoter of human rights conventions, knew they were interpersonal.

> Where, after all, do universal human rights begin? In small places, close to home – so close and so small that they cannot be seen on any maps of the world. Yet they are the world of the individual person … Such are the places where every man, woman, and child seeks equal justice, equal opportunity, equal dignity without discrimination. Unless these rights have meaning there, they have little meaning anywhere … Without concerted citizen action to uphold them close to home, we shall look in vain for progress in the larger world.[53]

The third real level concerns why rights matter as a driving force through history since, for example, the Jewish people left slavery in Egypt and journeyed to the Promised Land. Whether their eighth-century BCE *Exodus* was history or myth, it celebrates age-old hopeful protest against oppression and injustice.[54] The common people's demands for justice have gradually been refined, from the seventeenth century onwards, by philosophers and lawyers into modern empirical concepts of specific rights that make governments accountable.[55] Modern human rights express everyone's deep need for liberty, equality, solidarity and dignity, the grounds for physical, mental and social health.

Rights are sometimes dismissed as selfish individualism, but they are the opposite.

> A Declaration of Rights is, by reciprocity, a Declaration of Duties also. Whatsoever is my right as a man [*sic*] is also the right of another; and it becomes my duty to guarantee, as well as to possess.[56]

To claim a right involves recognising everyone's equal claim to that right, knowing that

> recognition of the inherent dignity and of the equal and inalienable rights of all members of the human family is the foundation of freedom, justice and peace in the world, Whereas disregard and contempt for human rights have resulted in barbarous acts which have outraged the conscience of mankind, and the advent of a world in which human beings shall enjoy freedom of speech and belief and freedom from fear and want has been proclaimed as the highest aspiration of the common people ...[57]

Rights involve everyone being able to choose to help and support others, not being forced to do so. Instead of dividing and reducing wellbeing in zero-sum ways, many rights multiply wellbeing in win-win ways. Clean air and water, good healthcare and justice systems benefit everyone. Epidemics spread more quickly when people do not have free healthcare services or sick pay benefits so that they must work or starve and therefore cannot stay at home.[58] Although they are often dismissed as 'Western' and not universal, human rights support movements around the world to defend and promote the wellbeing of individuals and groups. Gracelyn Smallwood showed through CR analysis how they relate to indigenous Australians, and potentially to all oppressed and colonised minorities.[59]

Following Marx, critical realists claim that the flourishing of each person depends on the flourishing of all, when no one can flourish if this is at the cost of other people's suffering. The view has been criticised as being too vague about the meaning of flourishing.[60] However the UN rights treaties spell out the basic adequate standards of living that everyone needs if they are to flourish. These make power1 rights real and compelling. Rights are countered by real power2 forces of selfish individuals' greed and ambition to conquer and control through cruelty and fear. Societies prevent such abuses when they require their governments to respect equal human rights. The growing impact of the climate crisis and of pandemics makes the above UDHR warning about 'barbarous acts' ever more urgent. Central to rights is respect for dignity.

Dignity

Debates on dignity are confused. Some treat dignity as an inner quality, an inherent part of being human, or at least of being a mature rational person. Alternatively, dignity is an external quality shown in the way others treat that person. Laura Valentini argues that:

> human rights are often defined as entitlements that human beings possess just by virtue of their inherent dignity. This conceptual link between human rights and inherent dignity is as popular as it is unhelpful to the core function of human rights: placing constraints on powerful actors, especially states. [Human rights are better served] by distinguishing between 'inherent dignity' and 'status dignity', and by linking human rights to the latter, not the former.[61]

This view raises complex questions about why certain people but not others should have human rights, and therefore why anyone should have rights at all. Also, why do the most vulnerable groups, and those in greatest need of respectful protection, tend to be most excluded from being rights-holders? They include all children or at least younger ones, besides people with severe learning difficulties, or dementia, or those who are comatose.

Again CR concepts of reality can help to clarify these uncertainties. The CR empirical level concerns individuals' views of dignity, their own and other people's, and their experiences of their dignity being respected or disrespected The bioethicist Ruth Macklin dismissed dignity as 'a useless concept' because of its irrelevance to how a corpse is treated: a corpse 'is no longer a person but a cadaver'.[62] Yet this denies the importance in most societies of respect for deceased people and their remains, celebrated in Sophocles's fifth-century BCE *Antigone*. And adults and children immediately know when their dignity is disrespected.

At the actual level of practical interactions, dignity and rights may be most apparent if they are ignored and people are abused, coerced, exploited or ridiculed. Without respect for patients' dignity, healthcare risks turning into a mechanical exercise without real motive, meaning or relationships. Morality then turns into rule-bound ethics, self-interested legal-economic precautions against patients making complaints, without real concern for their needs. Respect for healthcare professionals (pre-2020) was declining. The British government stopped collecting data on assaults against NHS staff in 2016, but research by their trade union Unison estimated there were more than 56,435 physical assaults on NHS staff in 2016–17.[63] When staff are underpaid and overworked, with too little time to care for patients to the standards everyone hopes to maintain, mutual respect between staff and patients is eroded.

At the real ontological level, dignity may be analysed as a causal power that impels and informs activities. The UN's themes mentioned earlier of 'the inherent dignity and of the equal and inalienable rights of all members of the human family' have been discussed, enshrined and ratified by governments across the world.[64] We are sentient, sapient, moral, social beings. Over millennia, natural selection appears to have favoured sociable caring human parents and babies. They enjoy higher rates of survival, so that mutual empathy and respect appear to have evolved into innate human capacities.[65] Morality that respects and cares for others can be learned and refined over the lifetime, but it is not synthetic, or wholly acquired or taught through words. Human morality and dignity have deeper foundations in being 'inherent', 'inalienable' and fused with innate human nature.

Margaret Archer analysed how our preverbal learning emerges through our biological body-brain and experience in the natural world.[66] From birth, babies interact with other people and react sensitively to their moods, happy, calm, anxious or angry. Within the first months, long before they can talk, babies begin to show moral awareness, detected through micro-video-recordings of their gaze and heartbeat rate.[67] That this moral capacity seems to be unique to human beings is one basis for respecting their inalienable dignity. It is part of learning from babies how to nurture their wellbeing and prevent their suffering.[68] The critical realist Christian Smith considers that dignity is emergent when persons can realise their *telos*. This is Aristotle's concept of individuals' purpose or goal, which is 'an inherent worth of immeasurable value that is deserving of certain morally appropriate responses'.[69]

Ineffable dignity, one's own and others', is empirically and subjectively experienced but also objectively and actually recognised, respected or disrespected. At actual and empirical levels, dignity may be ignored or seen as ephemeral and even imaginary. It therefore also needs to be understood at the unseen real level of causal mechanisms, at the default centre of human identity and relationships.[70]

Truth, trust and consent

At the empirical level, we often misunderstand or misrepresent truth and can only ever partly know it. At the actual level, people mislead others, practitioners deceive patients, politicians secretly privatise the NHS. Our daily experiences can suggest there is no such thing as truth, or only many versions of it. When social constructionists believe that everything emerges from and makes meaning within local contexts, they cannot accept universal truths. Yet as noted earlier, this leads to theory/practice inconsistency when researchers mistrust participants' accounts but expect their own reports to be believed. Interpretivist, contingent and relativist views of truth raise profound problems.

Natural necessity (the actual, empirical and real) aids analysis of the different levels of trust, truth and consent. Besides being distinct, the three levels overlap and interact. With health and illness, they can be understood through:

1. empirical ways in which people feel, think and talk about health;
2. the actual nature of trustful/mistrustful, truthful/deceptive, consenting/coercing relationships, interactions and discussions during practitioner-patient encounters; and
3. trust, truth and voluntary consent (which includes commitment and courage)[71] as real, powerful, unseen forces that influence people's beliefs and behaviours. Manipulation, deception and abuse of power are also causal mechanisms.

Truth is the default that we constantly rely on in everything. We assume the truth when walking down stairs of wood or stone that they will bear our weight. We will not sink into them as if they are like treacle. When we turn on a tap, we feel certain water will pour out, not acid. Reading this book is pointless unless you assume that I intend to write the truth, although I can only understand it partly and fallibly. And deception can only be defined in relation to how it deviates from enduring truth. Multilayered trust, such as in patient-doctor relations, includes cognitive trust based on rational practical information and personal trust based on intuition, emotions and empathic relationships.[72]

The CR view of truth challenges relativism. The ideals of voluntary consent and perfect truth and trust are seldom if ever fully achieved at empirical and actual levels. They might seem to be unrealistic illusions, perhaps better dispensed with in modern scientific medicine. Yet, like gravity in their enduring reality, they are like a compass, pointing towards the magnetic power of ideal trust and truth. These are unreachable, but they guide, define and evaluate all our interactions, in how nearly we approach them or how far we deviate from them. Trust, truth, and willingness or voluntariness are vital aspects of consent for practical useful reasons. They also matter at deep levels of our inalienable, authentic human nature. Table 4.1 summarises these sections on human rights, dignity, trust and truth.

Table 4.1: Natural necessity: rights, dignity, trust and truth

	Rights	Dignity	Trust	Truth
Empirical and local beliefs about how they are understood and respected or not	✓	✓	✓	✓
Actual practices that honour or violate them	✓	✓	✓	✓
Human needs and impulses that rely on these powerful universal default causal influences	✓	✓	✓	✓

Values in health research

Values concern what we most prize or value. They centrally involve physical wellbeing and survival. Benjamin Pauli connected our essential healthcare need for clean water to the values of social justice and the need for democratic, accountable public officers.[73] After their household water began to be supplied from a new source, residents in Flint, Michigan, soon found that the new supplies were contaminated with high levels of lead. Their struggle for safe affordable water became part of a broader struggle for democracy. Some citizens became 'water warriors'. They demanded that the elected officials be restored, with an end to the unaccountable appointed 'emergency managers'. The protestors expanded the struggle for water justice into a movement for a radically democratic Flint and a city of environmental justice. They showed how real values matter deeply, are passionately held and often relate to basic needs for health and survival. Conflicts over values can be long and bitter when each side is campaigning for what they most value (for the city authorities this was power and profit).

Sayer contends that critical social science (CSS) has become timid and cautious when it simply uncovers hidden presuppositions and deepens reflexivity.[74] The growing dichotomies, science/ethics, positive/normative, have diminished critical research, Sayer believes. He advocates that CSS works in three value-informed ways:

1. to reduce illusions and denaturalise social forms, by challenging assumptions that things are given, fated and inevitable, and by showing how alternatives are possible;
2. to assess and more clearly define freedom and flourishing and
3. to critique avoidable suffering.

On the example of freedom, Sayer considers that too often its complexities are overlooked. Notions of freedom are empty if they deny how we are all vulnerable and interdependent. Some of our major constraints are part of the most fulfilling aspects of our lives, caring for our family, for example. And to achieve anything, we have to work within necessary conditions.[75] Sayer finds the capabilities approach developed by Sen and Nussbaum useful for understanding complex freedoms.[76]

Nussbaum includes in her list, being able to have good health. This standard could exclude the estimated one billion disabled people,[77] besides countless others who are ill. Many of them flourish in spite of, or even because of, their difficulties. The notion would exclude deaf Beethoven, John Keats dying of TB, Marie Curie being poisoned by her radiation research and many other creative people during their active lifetime. Critical disabled researchers have transformed concepts of disability away from the medical model of problems within the person into the social model of disabling problems in social structures, such as public transport and buildings.[78] Activists posted photos of themselves in the 1990s holding up the traffic when they parked their wheelchairs in front of London buses. Today buses and buildings across the world have wheelchair access because of the powerful protests. They proved how access to an active social life and to work and study can greatly improve disabled and ill individuals' wellbeing and prosperity.

Haben Girma defines disability as an opportunity for innovation and shows how it can be a catalyst.[79] A human rights lawyer and disability advocate, she was the first deaf-blind Harvard law graduate. She emphasises that we are all interdependent. When she was 15 she went to Mali to help to build a school. She has learned non-visual techniques for everything from dancing salsa to handling an electric saw. She developed a text-to-braille communication system that enables her to have normal speed conversations. This was demonstrated in her radio interview.[80]

Yet the disabled critical realist Tom Shakespeare warns against overplaying the social construction of disability.[81] That can ignore how illness, impairments, mental health problems and learning difficulties do limit people's everyday life. It could discourage them and everyone else from arranging for the help they need. It could slide towards relativism. Power2 relations have real independent effects on health, although they can be challenged and changed. Shakespeare contends that the social model of disability is a tool, not a theory.[82] It is effective against social oppression, discriminatory cultural discourse and practical environmental barriers. It has raised the confidence and the practical inclusion of people with impairments and has worked well in many ways. Shakespeare considers disability is produced through the interaction between individual bodies and social environments.

Research about disability and illness must take account of political-economic contexts and values, such as how and why governments restrict sickness and disability benefits.[83]

Human rights could offer firmer grounds than capabilities for defining values and the good life, what to avoid and what to promote. Rights have evolved over centuries through practical mass struggle and suffering, besides intense expert and international debate. The lawyer Conor Gearty sees human rights as 'the ethical architecture necessary to decent everyday life ... the only contemporary idea with true universal and progressive appeal [in today's] post-socialist, post-religious haze of market supremacy'.[84] International rights enshrine the values that respect everyone's dignity. They do so through structures of accountability to an independent rule of law and, especially, equality. Nevertheless, Sayer's analysis shows how values matter and are central to any research about problems and potential remedies.[85] 'To say why anything warrants critique we need some conception of well-being and ill-being' in concepts pervaded by values.[86]

Roy Bhaskar, who was disabled in his later years, with Berth Danermark discussed how CR is doubly inclusive in disability research.[87] It can explore

> the exact nature of the determinations [of disability] and their interactions to be empirically determined case by case. And it ... [can apply] the insights of the other [research theories] while avoiding their drawbacks. [CR can be clearer and broader] than the other positions [about] the appropriate direction and context of explanatory research

and it avoids reductionism by working at several levels of reality.[88]

As previous chapters have shown, one CR strength is explicit analysis of metatheory or paradigm: specific assumptions about the nature of the objects studied (ontology) and the conditions of knowing about them (epistemology). Metatheories are too often tacitly and subconsciously assumed. Bhaskar and Danermark critically analysed metatheories applied in health research. They proposed a layered system of research that connects all aspects of disability: (i) physical, (ii) biological including physiological, medical or clinical, (iii) psychological, (iv) psycho-social, (v) socio-economic, (vi) cultural and (vii) normative kinds of influencers, context and effects.[89] They also attended to contexts and scale from micro to global and showed how the four planes of social being,[90] open systems and other CR concepts and frameworks can be helpful. They illustrated the levels with the case of Emma and her eating disorder, showing how 'this is the easiest way to do science and the only way to do it consciously and consistently'. Metatheories determine what we can and cannot know, such as when values are excluded or included. CR assumes that health can only be understood when values are taken into account in the aim to move from coercive power2 towards creative power1.[91]

Social research about health and illness, particularly qualitative research, tends to be seen as inferior to clinical research. Social theories, methods, reliability and outcomes and therefore their influence on healthcare policies and practices are all less respected. Clinical research has far more funding support and more prestigious journals than social research. Yet in reality, patients' social experiences are vital before, during and after their clinical treatment. Their social views and experiences weave into their physical or mental health, the causes and symptoms of their illnesses, their treatment and recovery or failure to recover.

This is clearly shown in the extreme example of the Charlie Gard case.[92] Doctors wanted to end mechanical ventilation of the baby when they believed he either lacked all awareness or else could be aware only or mainly of discomfort if not suffering. Charlie's parents wanted mechanical ventilation to continue. A series of court hearings, which hinged on beliefs about his quality of life, ended with Charlie being moved to a hospice where ventilation was withdrawn. A report by doctors noted the need,[93] besides for medical support, for attention to social aspects of doctor-child-parent relations, with clear responses to early minor difficulties before they grow into major ones. Parents who want to avoid contact with certain staff were given as one example. The medical authors of the report, however, did not mention systemic social and cultural structures within intensive care units. These include the striving to save life, to advance treatments and to sustain hope. The report, mainly by doctors, considered the effects rather than causes of the structural problems. Partly for good reasons, these aspiring social structures increase the difficulties for healthcare professionals and parents when they decide whether or not to 'let go' and agree to end seemingly futile treatment. Values in social structures and relationships have to be researched if the ethical problems in healthcare relationships are to be understood and prevented or resolved.

Ethics and health research, what can critical realism add?

Ethics and values have effectively been removed from being a central and substantive concern of much social research and reduced to a weak set of rules about research procedures.[94] Ethics has been partly outsourced and condensed into legal and administrative technical standards for research methods and protocols, vetted by research ethics committees (RECs) and institutional review boards (IRBs). Instead of learning from philosophers as they used to do, up to around 2000, REC-IRB members tend to be trained by administrators in ticking boxes. Yet ethics actually pervades every stage of research from first plans to final dissemination and impact.[95] CR shows how ethics and values are central to research topics and methods and need to be examined critically and explicitly.[96]

During the 1970s, the new specialty of bioethics that combines philosophy and law was developed to assist medical researchers.[97] They faced growing complaints about their sometimes dangerous exploitative research,[98] with new demands that they should request informed consent from their research subjects.[99] Bioethicists interpreted moral philosophy traditions of deontology from Aristotle to Kant, and of utilitarianism. They identified four universal principles: justice, respect for autonomy, non-maleficence (do no harm) and a lesser principle of beneficence (doing good).[100] Bioethics is informed by Kant's categorical imperative of respect for self-determination or autonomy: always treat persons as ends in themselves (authors of their own lives), never as the means to other people's ends.[101] Researchers, however, need to use participants if they are to conduct research.

Bioethics emerged from reactions to the Holocaust and has stressed individual autonomy and consent.[102] It has neglected distributive justice, social contexts and the global community,[103] as well as discriminations and racism, omissions that social researchers working with bioethicists could do much to redress.[104]

Bioethics upholds respect for informed and voluntary consent, which transforms people from being exploited research subjects into being informed, altruistic participants.[105] Current and recent violations by researchers prove the need to respect consent. For example, in a World Health Organization randomised control trial (RCT) in Malawi, Ghana and Kenya, during 2019–21, the vaccine Mosquirix has been administered to 720,000 children. The researchers said they rely on 'implied consent' and families are not told about the risks. The risks include a ten times higher rate of meningitis, increased cerebral malaria cases and doubling of female mortality among children who have the vaccine. Bioethicists commented: 'The failure to require informed consent is a serious breach of international ethical standards' and 'implied consent is no consent at all. We have no assurance that parents in fact received information about the study let alone that they understood it.'[106] After a trial with similar problems in Kenya, families waited through 15 years of legal battles before being paid small compensation after their children died or suffered from disabling meningitis.[107] Informed consent protects researchers and participants from the dangers of these low standards.

In the bioethics tradition of utilitarianism, utility has been defined as 'that property in any object, whereby it tends to produce benefit, advantage, pleasure, good, or happiness ... [or] to prevent the happening of mischief, pain, evil, or unhappiness to the party whose interest is considered'.[108] The concern to avoid pain and maximise pleasure involves serving majority groups.[109] While deontologists look back towards rights and duties agreed by past authorities, utilitarians look forward to the outcomes of their chosen actions. Utilitarianism raises problems when it is assumed that the ends justify the means. Highly valued ends (a cure for cancer) may excuse cruel research. The aim to serve the majority can risk harming minorities. Utilitarian questions about 'what works?' can turn into cost-benefit equations that could override rights and principles of freedom and justice.[110] Functionalist utilitarianism dominates today's bioethics. Deontology also raises dilemmas when 'doing good' may mean obeying rules that are harsh and unjust to certain individuals and groups. This especially affects research, when participants undertake the risks and future patients might benefit if the findings are published and implemented.

A third growing interest among bioethicists is virtue ethics,[111] again inspired by Aristotle but with less deontological emphasis on duties and more concern with pondering the good life and the good person.[112] Virtue is seen as a character trait, not a single action, learned through practising virtuous habits. Plato's 4 cardinal virtues are wisdom, justice, fortitude and temperance.[113] Aristotle's 18 virtues are each a golden mean between extremes: courage avoids either fear or recklessness, modesty avoids either shame or shamelessness. Virtue ethics has influenced capability theory,[114] which shares with CR the values of theory-practice consistency, practical moral wisdom and eudaimonia or the well-lived life and flourishing. There is also concern with being virtuous (ontology) rather than with more superficially discussing virtues (epistemology). In the eudaimonic society, 'each is true to, of, in and for themselves and every other (including future generations and other species) subject to the constraints imposed by nature'.[115]

Ethics involves much debated uncertainties. For example, can and should virtuous persons be trusted and granted much discretion and power to decide on moral questions? How can disagreements about virtuous decisions be resolved? Virtue ethics has been sexist in the past, and it risks being relativist when prized virtues vary so much between different cultures. It is not clear how rigorously virtues and ensuing decisions should be explained and accounted for.

However Philip Hérbert's lifelong work, with Wayne Rosen, of striving to be a good doctor highlights the importance of habitual virtues in each doctor's personal relationship with each patient: listening, respecting their views, keeping their secrets, truth-telling, helping not harming, admitting error, trying to decide what is right during each ethical difficulty and searching for common values in discussions with patients. The idea of the good doctor and nurse is tested, discussed and explained in the book through complicated cases that pose tough questions. Besides skill and knowledge, the authors recommend most highly the virtuous habits of compassion, prudence, altruism, trustworthiness and humility.[116] Perhaps not all practitioners would agree with this list, though perhaps most patients might agree with it. Table 4.2 summarises the above review of the three main versions of ethics within the three CR levels of reality.

Table 4.2: CR levels of reality and ethics

CR levels	Deontology	Utilitarianism	Virtue ethics
Empirical beliefs	Universal duties and principles	Cost-effectiveness and efficiency measures	Moral beliefs and emotions
Actual practices	Enacted duties	Follow rules and evidence to benefit majority	Virtuous habits, interactions and relations
Real causal influencers	Need and longing for justice, respect, avoiding harm	Need to promote pleasure and avoid pain, control costs and standards	Need and longing for the good life

Each tradition in bioethics raises vital moral questions for health research. They can thereby increase healthcare researchers' understanding of the benefits and problems in their work and the ways to analyse the related moral dilemmas. These include protecting vulnerable participants but not excluding them from research and balancing their interests with potential gains for society and for future patients. This summary about research ethics will end with a CR review of the responses to bioethics from different health research paradigms.[117]

Health research paradigms and ethics

Routine REC-IRB review of medical research protocols began from around 1980.[118] Yet routine review of social research was not formally advised in Britain until 2003.[119] Medical researchers tend to be more concerned about ethics than social researchers are.[120] This is possibly because medical research can cause more direct and obvious harm and therefore needs more protection from complaints and litigation, which REC-IRB review can offer. It may also be that doctors have greater control over bioethics systems than social researchers tend to have.[121]

Since the 1980s, REC-IRB review gradually became more efficient. It has helped to stop abusive research and to raise standards of respect for research participants and their informed consent or refusal. Yet through the 2010s, and since GDPR,[122] many ethics reviews in Britain and other countries have been severely delayed, wasting tens of thousands of pounds of funded research time.[123] Teams of administrators check and recheck and duplicate one another's work and demand copious paperwork.[124] Some social researchers criticise research ethics, and their key comments are summarised here.[125]

- There is rivalry between the social sciences and bioethics, and concern that review systems informed by bioethics and law have too much power and too little knowledge of social science.
- REC-IRB review can be very costly, absorbing precious research time and funds. It may incur 'the diversion of resources; the promotion of ignorance; and the stifling of innovation'.[126] Valuable projects may be misjudged, delayed, reduced or rejected.
- Medical research needs careful ethical protections, but does social health research, since it does not incur the same dangers?
- Ethics regulation is designed to protect powerful institutions (hospitals, universities), their reputations and income, rather than to support social research or participants.
- Academic freedom is compromised. One critic was 'outraged' to see that 'Conducting research is a privilege and NOT a right.'[127]

These are all important points, but they raise problems. In reply to the final point, researchers' right to freedom of thought and enquiry is sacrosanct. Yet when researchers rely on funders and participants, researchers' rights are not absolute but are qualified to respect the other people concerned. Harms to patients are more than physical; their suffering is primarily social.[128] Social research can seriously harm individual participants by causing anxiety, shame or loss of privacy. If flawed research 'evidence' supports inefficient or abusive services, it can harm whole groups. Pre-1970s research tended to be sexist, racist, colonialist and prejudiced against disabled people and other minority groups. Might today's more respectful, humane and inclusive research have been encouraged by the ethics review system?

'But perhaps the real source of our ethical dilemma is that we do not – or perhaps no longer – believe that ethics committees "do ethics" in the way that we as social scientists think ethics needs to be done in practice.'[129] More informed debate is needed between social scientists and ethicists.

CR can contribute the first steps, with immanent critique of how social research theories can open or close vision and insight into ethics. 'Value-free' positivists may ignore how their objective impersonal paradigm attempts to exclude ethics along with other values. For example, ANT researchers may deny ethical aspects of their research, when they do not recognise moral agents or 'the first-person, action-guiding character of morality'.[130] Relativist interpretivists' belief only in limited, contingent versions of ethics rejects REC-IRB support for universal ethics. International researchers may assume RECs-IRBs are biased and are only relevant to one country or locality. CR counters these positivist and relativist views. CR contends that ethics and values have real, potentially universal, causal meaning and power, although these cannot be fully known or understood and are interpreted and practised in varying ways.[131]

The critics' sharp dichotomies reject boundary-crossing movements. However, CR supports the critical creative interdisciplinary and international exchange being developed by many researchers.[132] One proposal is 'a methodology of the heart, a performative, indigenous, feminist, communitarian ethic that embraces an ethics of truth grounded in love, care, hope, and forgiveness'.[133] Most researchers support ethicists' universal principles, at least in practice in their personal lives if not in theory. This is despite difficulties applying them in practice since 'context, history, culture, and politics, as well as the social, gender, and economic status of participants, can have implications for how ethical principles are applied in different settings'.[134] There is support for feminist, critical, postcolonial and Indigenous reports to inform REC-IRB members' capacity-building in international ethics.[135] An 'Afro-communitarian' notion of mutuality, *ubuntu*, might be better suited to research in sub-Saharan Africa than an imported ethics of care.[136] High-income counties can learn from low-income ones.[137] CR can deepen understanding of ethics generally and of complex ethical dilemmas, such as whether to separate conjoined twins when only one could survive.[138]

After working with bioethicists for decades, with some tensions, the sociologist Renée Fox called for deeper interdisciplinarity with them.[139] This would be: more philosophical; less reductive and trapped in dichotomies; more involved in clinical and policy spheres; more seriously engaged with human suffering, relationships and personhood; more aware and respectful of cultural differences within and between societies and of global social justice and poverty. CR supports this interdisciplinary concern with ontology and with connecting many aspects of complex ethics in research, beginning with the analysis of tacit research theories and paradigms that may block progress. Table 4.3 is a CR summary of this section on the views about ethics in different research paradigms.

Table 4.3: Research paradigms and views of ethics

	Interpretivism	Positivism	CR
Empirical	Analyse context-bound ethical beliefs and standards	Keep ethics within methods	Respect ethical beliefs and standards in methods and substance of research
Actual		Objective records and measures of ethics-related events	Subjective and objective being and doing of ethics, values, virtues; actual suffering and flourishing
Real			Inalienable ethical values, needs, rights and aspirations

Ethical naturalism and moral realism

CR ethical naturalism assumes that human life and human nature are inevitably imbued with integral morality. Researchers do not add or impose an external morality into their work. Instead, realistic research explores the central morality in all social life. The aim is to discover what really matters and to search for and reveal unethical beliefs and practices, and find alternatives.[140]

An example is Rosa Mendizabal's neonatal research.[141] She documented unethical routines that contradicted the practitioners' claim that these served the babies' wellbeing. She checked how the local rules might be necessary or preferable in Mexican hospitals but could not find evidence to support them. She assessed the Mexican standards against her experience in a humane, 'baby-led', well-resourced London NICU. She followed CR explanatory critique, which:

1. identifies problems – unmet needs, suffering and false beliefs;
2. identifies the source or cause of those problems;

3. passes to a negative judgement of those sources of illusion and oppression and
4. favours actions that remove those sources.[142]

Moral realism sees morality, human rights, justice, freedom and compassion as all having an 'objective real property' and enduring existence.[143] Although their detailed meanings are contested, and they are experienced and practised in many different ways, their core, underlying, universal reality can be known powerfully; see Table 4.3. Real causal influences include the human impulses to promote values, avoid suffering and increase wellbeing.[144]

The positivist idea, 'of social factors in health and disease … from which the policy implications will flow',[145] was cited in Chapter 2. Science does not impersonally produce policy, as the 2020 SAGE advisers showed. Reported evidence may be promoted, ignored or misused by policymakers, whose choices are influenced by expedience, funding, powerful personalities, rival interest groups and party politics. Researchers' beliefs that they are 'unbiased' ignore their choices throughout research, from first plans and funding applications, to how and where to report their findings, within the political world of health research funders, sponsors, access to data and journal review.[146] Bambra and colleagues (non-CR, public health experts) advise that political science expertise is needed to enable health researchers to explain, for example, why health inequalities are occurring and increasing.[147]

Sayer questions the tenuous, sometimes arbitrary, links between evidence and policy. He calls

> for renewed discussion about the relationship between knowledge-based and value-based dimensions of decision-making … [which] requires a more circumspect and less fundamental role for knowledge of 'what works' than supporters of evidence-based policy are typically willing to allow. The epistemic emphasis of 'what works' discourse needs to be complemented and counterbalanced with greater appreciation of the value of conceptual clarity, public deliberation, local and experiential forms of knowledge.[148]

Learning from other major theorists: advocacy on many levels

One research approach to public health examines the politics and justice of class as a major determinant (causal mechanism) of health inequality.[149] Another less obviously value-influenced approach compares income inequality in different societies and associated health standards.[150] CR researchers tend to favour the first, more critical, approach and also to draw on work in other theories and disciplines. Example 4.1 links values, politics and CR to Habermas's class-based analysis of heartlessly destructive policies. There is reference to neoliberalism, which researchers often avoid as if it is both a biased and a vague term. Part of the triumph of neoliberalism is the frequent denial that it exists. Yet regimes like feudalism or capitalism have greater power if the label is denied or ignored, and they are seen as simply normal and TINA.[151] Another triumph of neoliberalism is that attempts at its alternatives, (real) communism or socialism, rarely succeed, or endure, or they are sabotaged and seen as dangerous corrupt failures.

Bourdieu defined neoliberalism as a programme for destroying any collective structures that may impede pure market logic.[152] David Harvey showed how neoliberalism takes market exchange as the model and guide for all human action.[153] To Naomi Klein and Philip Mirowski, neoliberals plunder and transform societies during natural or financial shocks and crises.[154] They commercialise healthcare, set private interests over public ones, cut many health-related state services and adversely affect the lives and health of millions of people.[155] Some public health researchers conclude that 'the obesity, insecurity, austerity and inequality that result from neoliberal (or "market fundamentalist") policies are hazardous to our health'. These neoliberal epidemics require a political cure.[156] Political themes in Example 4.1 will be developed further in Chapter 7.

Example 4.1: Combining critical realism with Habermas's theories

By Graham Scambler, University College London, UK

My work on the sociology of health, illness and healthcare has always been oriented to describing social phenomena and explaining why they are as they are. I have drawn on various philosophers and social theorists to assist in this process, my concern being less the faithful following of their leads than adapting and *using* their contributions for my own purposes. I shall concentrate in this brief précis on the critical realism of Roy Bhaskar and the critical theory of Jurgen Habermas and their salience for the study of long-term stigmatising conditions and health inequalities.

Bhaskar's philosophy of critical realism, at the core of which is his exposure and response to the 'epistemic fallacy', namely, the centuries-old tendency for philosophers to reduce 'what exists' (ontology) to 'what we (can) know of what exists' (epistemology). Taking my cue from his basic critical realism (BCR), I came to define my task as the retroductive and/or abductive inference to those social structures, cultures and modes of human agency that *must exist* given our understanding of those *events* made accessible to us through our *experience*. I ended up focusing in particular on the causal power of social structures, or relations, like those of class and state. Hence my exposure of the 'class/command dynamic' underpinning the genesis and widening of health inequalities in post-1970s financialised capitalism. According to this dynamic, a tiny fraction of the largely transnational capitalist executive has come to dominate the national command relations of the state, one unintended consequence of this being shifts in policy that have rendered the disadvantaged more vulnerable to poor health and premature death. Expressed as a formula: class-based capital buys power from the state to make policy that prioritises further capital accumulation. Health inequalities are collateral damage.

I deployed aspects of Bhaskar's dialectical critical realism (DCR) to deepen my BCR-rooted investigations. For example, I used his observation that being is but a ripple on the surface of the ocean of non-being to highlight the importance of the idea of *absence*. One general ramification of highlighting absence rather than being is that it brings into focus the pivotal but typically neglected insight that social phenomena like health inequalities, and the neoliberal ideology that presents them as the product of individual lifestyle choices, do not have to be as they are and might yet be transformed. More specifically, it exposes standard social scientific measurement proxies for (occupational) class as absenting any meaningful analysis of those class relations most pertinent to the class/command dynamic: in short, it absents that fragment of the 1 per cent that pulls the strings of the state, thus 'sheltering' our plutocracy or governing oligarchy from quantitative analysis.

Sticking with the themes introduced here, I also found the social theories of Habermas of value. Consider the class/command dynamic. Habermas' theory of strategic versus communicative action affords a new and rewarding frame for deepening the sociological analysis.[157] Habermas argues that modern Western societies have witnessed a de-coupling of the system (comprising economy and state and characterised by strategic or means/ends action and oriented to outcome) and the lifeworld (comprising the private and public spheres in which we act out our everyday private and public lives and characterised by communicative action oriented to consensus). This de-coupling has given rise to a system 'colonisation' of the lifeworld. On this reading, the class/command dynamic is one articulation of the system colonisation of the lifeworld.

An additional virtue of Habermas' system/lifeworld dichotomy is that it affords a ready opportunity to trace macro- to micro-social linkages. For example, exchanges between doctors and patients can be appraised in terms of the relative inputs of structurally based strategic versus communicative action. Consider a routine consultation in general practice. What Habermas calls open strategic action occurs when the GP straightforwardly asserts his or her expert knowledge and assumes, even requires, patient assent. More interesting is the concept of concealed strategic action. This can take two forms. Distorted communication constitutes a form of manipulation, for example, when the GP deliberately uses technical medical terms to intimidate, subdue or silence a patient narrative of interrogation or protest. Most interesting of all, however, is a second type of concealed strategic action, systematically distorted communication. This characterises an encounter when both GP and patient are acting in good faith, *and yet their dialogue and any decision-making arising out of it are indirect products of system colonisation*.

By way of illustrating this notion of systematically distorted communication, we can return to the class/command dynamic. I have argued that this is the principal causal mechanism for the widening gap in health inequalities. It is also, via the Health and Social Care Act of 2012 (H&SC Act), key to explaining the neoliberal undermining and privatisation of health services under the NHS brand. As Chomsky has argued, if you want to privatise a state institution you first starve it of resources, thereby creating public dissatisfaction, and then you appeal to the private sector to 'rescue it'. The NHS has been run down and private, for-profit healthcare companies at home and abroad are using the H&SC Act – largely under the radar – to take over services, including some in primary care. Thus it might be that while a GP and his or her patient *appear to be, and believe they are, interacting in good faith* they are in fact acting out system rationalising and lifeworld colonising scripts.

So in summary I have found a synthesis of Bhaskar's critical realist ontology and Habermas' critical theoretical framework for 'doing substantive/empirical sociology' fruitfully. I have, I hope, given a flavour of this from my work on health and healthcare. The post-1970s era of financialised capitalism has, I maintain, delivered a *fractured society* inimical to the material and social wellbeing of those already disadvantaged and, an aspect of this same process, foreshortened their lifespans.

Another useful example of Habermas' lifeworld theory is a study of the much encouraged Public and Patient Initiative.[158] When researchers ask participants to advise them, this can end in the research system colonising the participants' lifeworld responses. Participants then end up simply watching or supporting the researchers.[159]

Realist evaluation, critical realism and values

This final section returns to the critical debate between Ray Pawson (RE) and Samuel Porter (CR).[160] They debated values,[161] and Pawson claimed that RE is value-neutral. The fact/value distinction must be kept if RE is not to 'abandon analysis for ideology', which is the 'fundamental error' of CR.[162] Yet adopting values does not mean abandoning analysis, and realist evaluators themselves cannot avoid value judgements. Porter replied that RE researchers who claim to be 'value-free' risk reinforcing unjust inequalities.[163] Their 'uncritical approach ... combined with [the] underplaying of the importance of agency, leaves it open to implication in the abuses of bureaucratic instrumentalism,'[164] and other oppressive power. One example is when 'effective' is taken to mean 'cost-effective' rather than, say, patients' or nurses' views about humanely effective care. Another example is when health promotion means addressing patients' 'social problems' by trying to change their beliefs and behaviours instead of by challenging political or economic causes of their problems.[165] This can lead to dangerous victim-blaming.[166]

Porter contended that social scientists have the moral responsibility to acknowledge when their work 'often has real consequences for people [who have] value-laden concerns'. RE researchers accept that the social world is infinitely complex. Porter believes they should therefore make explicit transparent judgements about the inevitable values in their work. To 'hide behind the fig leaf of disinterested [value-free] science is false modesty'.[167] 'This is all the more important' given the 'significant public role ... of evidence-based policy and practice'.[168] RE's 'lack of robust critical values and the adherence to Popperian piecemeal social engineering' pushes 'technical solutions' that may be alienating.[169] This can transmute 'personal and ethical problems into scientific and technological categories ... [and it] devalues the lifeworlds.'[170] Realist evaluators claim they avoid the dangerous fanaticism of 'utopian social engineering',[171] to concentrate on 'what works for whom in what circumstances'.[172] Yet Porter considers that

CR's concern with holistic social progress and individual agency 'provides a solid guard against the slide into technocratic consciousness' that tinkers with piecemeal change.[173] CR relies on ethics centred on people's own concerns and experiences.

Summary

RE research about US Family-Nurse Partnership (FNP) programmes illustrates and connects value-related themes considered through this chapter and earlier ones. Large RCTs were designed to show the efficacy of FNP work 'to support vulnerable young parents'. The researchers used a GRADE system guided by efficacy and 'the value of utility'.[174] Their favoured term 'stakeholders' implied an equality that denies how unequal the power and the 'stakes' may be. Stakes include parents' fear that if they admit their serious problems their children will be taken from them into care.[175] Researchers investigated whether the US FNP model was more effective (cheaper with larger caseloads) than UK health visitor services. Promotion of cost-cutting services could waste money by reducing efficacy.

Missing information included: the parents' views; the effects of higher workloads on health visitors' anxiety that they will be disciplined or sacked if any child is seriously harmed; and how their anxiety affects their relations with parents. Many parents mistrust health visitors as 'agents of the state'.[176] This can undermine health visitors' main work in their nursing skills of helpful early intervention and health promotion, which depend on trusting relationships.[177]

In contrast to RE, CR research explicitly examines:

- values, power, politics and other unseen causal influences;
- how relationships and the collection, analysis and reporting of health research findings may be affected by trust, respect and equality, or their absence;
- how values, morals and rights inhere in human ontology, the being and doing of embodied experience, needs, hopes and relationships and
- absences and better future alternatives, not only past evidence (see Chapter 7).

Without 'a critical stance towards the values of policy makers, there is a danger that … there may be negative consequences for people that are not picked up by the evaluators'.[178] Everyone has concerns informed by their observations, reasoning and values, which are integral to facts about their lives and needs. Values do not mandate a particular response. They raise questions and discussions about how best to examine and relieve suffering and promote flourishing.[179]

The next two chapters consider ways to combine many aspects of our social-natural-moral lives instead of attempting to split them apart and set them in opposition. Chapter 5 is mainly about space, and levels from micro to macro, which were referred to in Example 4.1.

Questions to write or talk about with colleagues

1. What questions about values are raised by your research?
2. How do you address values, power, respect or trust in your research?
3. How do bioethics questions relate to the content as well as the methods of your research?
4. Does your research address moral personhood and dignity?
5. Can you think of any social facts that do not involve values?
6. Discuss how you could combine CR analysis with ideas from a major theorist who has influenced health and illness research (Example 4.1).

5

Four planes of social being: more connections

> There are high rates of cancer in Bayelsa State in the Niger Delta in an 'eco-genocide'.[1] Families drink toxic water and breathe toxic air. Children climb over great oil pipes on their way to school. For decades, multinational oil companies have left old pipes and machinery to leak oil into the rivers and across the land, destroying local wells, crops, herds and wildlife. Around 40 million litres of oil are spilled annually in the Niger Delta, in comparison to 4 million litres of oil spilled in the whole United States each year. It is estimated that oil spills could have killed around 16,000 babies within their first month of life. Life expectancy in the Niger Delta is about ten years lower than the national average.
>
> A Commission of Inquiry reviewed environmental, health, socio-economic, cultural and human damage and also identified unseen influences.[2] The Commission concluded that the oil companies put profit first. Their policies are racist and neo-colonialist when Nigerian lives in the delta are deemed to be worthless. The oil sales bring in 40 per cent of the GNP, which could deter government action to prevent pollution.[3] No national or international standards can be enforced to control the companies. The ten Commission members advised on a new legal framework to ensure accountability: the oil companies should agree to a global standard of behaviour and operate in Bayelsa as they would in Norway, Scotland or the USA.

The Inquiry's proposed remedy partly depends on the market reforming itself, and the Inquiry members seem to overlook further problems. These include vast investments in fossil fuel companies, such as by Western governments, pension funds and university endowments.[4] International financial trading system algorithms are set up to divert funds by the micro-second to the most profitable companies. Shareholders are supposed to hold companies to account and to see that they maintain reasonable standards. Yet shareholders' own first motive is profit, and this is their duty to the investors they represent. Shareholders also have almost no power over company policies. The decades of delay to reform will continue unless these barriers are addressed.

When researchers have collected huge amounts of data, perhaps like the Inquiry members, they may feel overwhelmed. Even if they use multivariate analysis, researchers face daunting questions about how to select, manage, analyse, interconnect and make sense of the many findings. Critical realism (CR) has useful frameworks to assist this analysis, such as the four planes of social being, which cover every aspect of being human. A first step may be to sort the data into these four planes, which can highlight and deepen understanding of all the constantly interacting levels of human life. Earlier chapters noted that large-scale quantitative research provides vital background information about health and healthcare. Yet it can lose sight of complex individual agency. Qualitative studies of individuals and small groups may over-emphasise agency and unusual examples, and they may not support valid general conclusions. CR methods of combining large- and small-scale studies to resolve these problems will be reviewed with examples.

This chapter considers CR approaches to managing data analysis: the four planes of social being; laminated systems analysis; interdisciplinary research and policymaking; CR theories about interdisciplinarity; overcoming barriers to interdisciplinarity and interdisciplinary commitments.

Four planes of social being

The four planes that cover every aspect of being human are: bodies in relation to nature; interpersonal relations; larger social relations and structures; and inner human being in the mental-social-embodied personality.[5] They are illustrated here by Kate Martin's doctoral research about young people's share in decision-making in psychiatric units. Martin began by thinking the first plane about bodies and nature was hardly relevant to her study.[6] Surely her concern was with minds, not bodies. Yet the first plane helped her to see the very unhealthy physical lifestyle that young people had to endure in the wards, how this was generally overlooked by the healthcare team and how bodies were actually central to her research. So too were the other three constantly interacting planes, as a framework of analysis.

At plane one, Martin observed the inactive daily life of the young people mainly shut indoors and their poor diet. Some medications intended to help their minds disturbed their bodies. During the weekly 'ward round', the staff did not walk round the wards. Instead, partly to protect privacy, they discussed the mainly absent patients in a separate office. The lack of their embodied presence and voice may have reinforced patients' lowly status in the hospital hierarchy and staff discussion on plane two. Senior psychiatrists and psychologists planned treatments that were mainly provided by junior nurses and assistants. When junior staff misunderstood or disagreed with prescribed behaviour treatments, such as to reduce obsessive compulsive disorder, they did not always enforce it. Lack of regular embodied and interpersonal contact between the young people and senior staff symbolised and may have reinforced a version of the epistemic fallacy: the consultants' view that ideas devised in 'ward rounds' are self-sufficient and can simply be imposed onto resistant patients and systems.

Many of the young people had severe problems, partly because they had to wait so long before they could receive treatment. Since 2010, austerity policies in Britain have cut mental health and youth and education services. They have increased the stressors,[7] such as long waiting lists for treatment, poverty, poor insecure crowded housing,[8] delays in universal credit payments for families, and school exclusions. There are also the 'hostile environment' towards perceived immigrants and the PREVENT counter-terrorism programme,[9] which greatly distress many ethnic minority young people. There is severe neglect of the most vulnerable children, including refugees and asylum seekers and looked-after children in unregulated children's homes. Loneliness and anxiety about bullying on social media have also very much increased. Health services need to be seen in these socio-economic contexts on the third plane of social being.

Inner being and psychological states are central to Martin's research on plane four. Archer's internal conversations aided her analysis of interviews with young people and staff in the units.[10] Young people in their interviews appeared to be rational and reflexive in Archer's first three groups: autonomous, communicative or meta-reflexive. Yet the staff tended to interpret the young people's views and behaviours as being in the fourth group: fractured reflexivity, irrational and untrustworthy. This opened Martin's analysis of how power and medicalising regimes construct irrationality when it does not always exist and so impede therapeutic relationships.

Many students base each of the four main chapters of their thesis or dissertation on a different plane of social being. It is not always possible to cover all the four planes in detail in a single research programme. Yet it is worth alluding to them all and showing awareness of their influences and effects. Methods of doing so include 'nesting' small-scale research inside multidisciplinary literature reviews or setting their context by referring to large surveys, systematic reviews, the geo-historical background or current policy and public debates.

Stuart Green Hofer's doctoral research also showed how the four planes help to cross boundaries and reveal new insights and connections in mental healthcare.

Example 5.1: Improving the physical health of people with a diagnosis of serious mental illness

Stuart Green Hofer, London School of Hygiene and Tropical Medicine, UK[11]

In the UK, life expectancy for people living with a diagnosis of serious mental illness (SMI) is reduced by 15–20 years compared with the general population.[12] This is primarily related to increased prevalence of respiratory, endocrine and circulatory disorders.[13] Despite existing evidence-based guidelines and policies, which indicate that acute mental health services should regularly assess the risk of this population through cardio-metabolic monitoring, this is poorly undertaken.[14]

My doctoral research explored the use of quality improvement as a participatory approach to bring together service users and healthcare professionals between 2014 and 2018.[15] Collectively, participants co-designed, implemented and scaled-up evidence-based interventions to support the improved assessment, communication and management of physical health within an acute mental health unit. I was both researcher and improvement facilitator, generating data through participant observations, documents and key informant interviews. The improvement team was able to improve and sustain physical health assessments, communication and delivery of interventions to prevent cardiovascular disease and diabetes and their complications[16]. However, my research focused on three underlying phenomena relating to quality improvement: mechanisms for navigating complexity to introduce improvements; the process of co-creating knowledge; and improvement as a social practice. This research used critical realism concepts, including the recognition that events simultaneously occur across four planes of social being. This concept of a laminated system represents the complexity of the social world, which can only be truly accounted for when understood across all four planes.

One example is the interaction between serious mental illness and physical health.

1. *Material relations of actors with nature* – could be understood as activities such as the consumption of high calorie/low nutrient food resulting in weight gain and activities such as smoking, drinking and taking drugs that exacerbate disease processes or medications that aim to modify these disease processes. These also include sedentary behaviour and an 'absence' of interaction with nature.
2. *Interpersonal subjective relationships* – highlight the role of health and social care professionals in both identifying and treating the presence of physical health conditions and risk factors for these conditions. Early identification and treatment are essential in ameliorating the long-term consequences of such conditions, which when left undiagnosed and untreated contribute to the early mortality of this population. So, while the absence of care may contribute to increased mortality, the treatments may also contribute to it. Support from the family and carers is also a key.
3. *Broader social relations and inherited social and institutional structures* – recognise the role of health and social care institutions in ensuring the physical wellbeing but also suggest the importance of broader determinants of health. These may include the relationships people with SMI have with their family or community and their impact of both positive and negative experiences. The fragmentation of these systems, especially where mental and physical health are both separated and perceived differently, may also affect their mental and physical health.
4. *Inner being – the stratified personality* – relates to the real choices that people with SMI are able to make to take control of their mental and physical health and their individual interpretation of wellbeing. While society, and healthcare in particular, may separate out mental and physical health, for the individual these are intricately and inseparably linked. The will to make lasting changes that can have positive effects has to come from within the individuals who need to feel empowered so they can express their agency to make decisions.

My research was developed to better understand some of the challenges encountered when implementing clinical guidelines, which have mainly been developed within a positivist epistemology. Through a critical realist lens, the analysis has highlighted the tensions that arise when attempting to understand the interplay between mental and physical health and allowed some of these complexities to emerge and co-exist. This is against a predominant view of the duality of their nature and separation of their understanding, which is deeply embedded in the human understanding and practice of healthcare.

Specifically, the four planes of social being highlight the complex nature of physical health within a mental health context. They recognise parts of the system that were not explored in previous research, which, for example, only really recorded healthcare professionals' practices. However, I was able to consider the views and experiences of people with a diagnosis of serious mental illness and the interactions between their physical and mental illness. Additionally, my research situated the quality improvement processes within this broader context and highlighted how they related to other aspects of the system, such as mechanisms for empowering patients.

On a more practical level, CR offers some understanding of how tensions within quality improvement methods simultaneously reinforce older structures and provide new spaces for healthcare professionals, service users and researchers to enact agency.

Laminated systems analysis

CR's laminated (layered) system also connects every level of human life from individuals' subconsciousness and genes to national and international structures, as shown in Example 5.2.

Example 5.2: Research into feminist-informed counselling after sexual assault

Bree Weizenegger, PhD Candidate, University of Melbourne, Australia[17]

Many victims-survivors of sexual violence experience post-traumatic stress symptoms.[18] Current evidence-based treatments include attempts to change individuals' neurobiological response of fear and avoidance, or their cognitive processing.[19] These treatments are based on reductive assumptions:[20] that problems of human distress exist and are caused within individuals' neurobiology but not in the socio-political context.[21] Although psychiatry and psychology purport to use bio-psycho-social models, this is rare.[22] 'As a profession, we have allowed the bio-psycho-social model to become the bio-bio-bio model.'[23] Psychiatrists and psychologists adopt the positivism of physical medicine (see Chapters 1 and 2). They search for causes of distress in biological correlations (DNA, genetics, neurons, neurotransmitters, brain scans) or in cognitive-behavioural ones (observations or reports on thoughts and behaviours). But human experiences, within complex relationships, social structures and open systems, cannot be reduced to biology and brains or correlations within closed systems.[24] How could the effects of colonisation on an aboriginal woman's experience of sexual assault be demonstrated? Such complex, immeasurable, invisible and un-knowable experiences need more holistic in-depth understanding. However, information from postmodern and interpretivist studies is not included in evidence-based treatment protocols for psychological distress.

Critical realism refutes the positivist confusion of correlations with causes and moves beyond the evidence-based paradigm to recognise and identify unseen causes in the complex real world (Chapter 2).The critical realist concept of a *laminated system* was important in my research.[25] The term 'laminated system' refers to the separate but interconnected strata in the reality of the specific time-and-place snapshots being studied (Table 5.1). Researchers may concentrate on only one of these strata, though it is important to see the full complexity of the open system. The strata connect feminist counselling to social justice, political analysis and geo-historical and macro forces on individuals' psychological and emotional experiences, which positivist research cannot do.[26]

Table 5.1: Laminated system for psychological research into distress

Level	This research
Geo-historical	Patriarchy, capitalism, racism, ableism
Macro	Australian medical, mental health and legal systems
Structural-meso	Relational positioning between: service user and counsellor/advocate counsellor/advocate and employer
Micro-social	Interaction between: service user and counsellor/advocate service user and supports counsellor/advocate and colleagues
Sub-individual	
Individual	Biography of service users and counsellors/advocates
Psychological	Thoughts, beliefs, desires, fantasies, values and reasons
Emotional	Unconscious and conscious emotional sensations and experiences
Physiological	Whole-of-body experiences and disease
Biological	Neurons, synapses, hormones

Source: Model adapted from Bhaskar and Danermark, 2006

Although similar to bio-psycho-social models such as Bronfenbrenner's ecological systems theory,[27] the CR laminated system recognises ontology: the different strata emerge from one another, but they are distinct from one another and are *irreducible*.[28] Although the brain, the mind, a human being and a society are interconnected and co-constitutive, we cannot hope to explain or understand the upper strata (a human person) by regressing to the lower strata (neurons).

An understanding of neurons cannot explain why a woman feels betrayed and ashamed after her parents blame her for being sexually assaulted. Sometimes, we need a 'macro regress' to the structures an individual is embedded in to more fully understand and address human distress.[29] The psychological science concepts of a flat ontology are too limited to research wider causes of human suffering and can only produce treatment options of medication or cognitive therapy. Crucially, understanding causes of human distress through laminated systems and complex open systems brings new ways to alleviate that distress.

Feminist counselling recognises that much human distress is caused by power and its abuse and by structures and systems that devalue and discriminate against many oppressed groups.[30] However, because these are rarely acknowledged, many individuals can only understand or explain their suffering in terms of the self: I am mad, I am bad, I am lazy, I am to blame. In the case of child sexual abuse and adult sexual assault, self-blame and the associated shame are high.[31] An intra-psychic approach to adult sexual assault, dominant in the psychological sciences, is to call self-blame a kind of cognitive distortion,[32] an attribution style,[33] or a way to maintain belief in the just nature of the world.[34] All these explanations assume the problem is with the individual's processing. In a patriarchal society with a dominant rape culture, doubting or blaming a sexual assault victim and excusing a sexual assault perpetrator is the norm.[35] Is a victim-survivor's self-blame a cognitive distortion in such a society or is it an expected outcome in the way adopting native languages and cultural practices also is?

A feminist analysis would explain victim-survivors' self-blame as being influenced by rigid gender roles within a sexist society.[36] This is a 'macro regress' to more fully understand a 'micro' phenomenon. But when macro forces cause human suffering, how can different treatment at the micro level address them? My research examined this question in feminist-informed sexual assault counselling. I used participant interviews and empirical, clinical and interpretivist literature from the feminist, trauma, sexual assault and sociological literature. I identified mechanisms within the counselling that addressed and ameliorated victim-survivors' experiences of self-blame. One of these mechanisms was a shift in consciousness for victim-survivors, from their original belief that they could have prevented the sexual violence to an understanding that they did not have the power to prevent the sexual violence. This shift in consciousness followed discussions in counselling regarding power dynamics between the perpetrator and the victim and the place of rigid gender roles in perpetuating myths about responsibility for sexual violence.

Wider concepts of a complex social system in which human beings are embedded – rather than simplifying complexity down to neurobiology – and the possibility to explore and discover causation within this complex system – rather than just empirical correlation – is possible due to critical realism's laminated ontology. This offers a viable and superior theory to investigate the causation and alleviation of human psychological and emotional distress.

Interdisciplinary research and policymaking

Among the many interdisciplinary research teams, think-tanks and review panels, one is conducting a comprehensive scientific five-year analysis of inequalities of income, wealth, health, social mobility, political participation and more. The aim is to understand the causes of inequalities and propose concrete policies to reduce them.[37] The panel that oversees and commissions the research programme plans to combine rigour with attention to people's everyday experiences. It 'includes world-leading experts in sociology, epidemiology, political science, philosophy and economics'. They consider that some inequalities are inevitable but that great inequalities of income or opportunity or health can disrupt democracy and prosperity. Rules and systems need to be changed in everyone's interests.

The review chair, economist Angus Deaton, warned that the UK should avoid some models set by the US. With Anne Case, he has researched how flaws in capitalism are fatal for America's working class, wherein (before the COVID-19 pandemic) over 150,000 middle-aged people died each year from suicide, drug overdose and alcoholism.[38] Since 2014, average American life expectancy has declined for the first time since records began in 1933. Deindustrialisation, stagnating wages and family breakdown tear apart once secure stable communities. They are prey to extremely costly private healthcare providers and to the opioid epidemic. Case and Deaton consider both these major health hazards are iatrogenic:[39] doctors are responsible for greatly overcharging patients and for years of mass over-prescribing of the addictive and mainly ineffective opioid painkillers. US college-educated adults become healthier and wealthier each year, while many other adults are dying in pain and despair.

Case and Deaton conclude that capitalism, which over two centuries lifted countless people out of poverty, is now destroying the lives of blue-collar Americans. They wanted to turn from the current US model towards solutions that can rein in capitalism's excesses and make it work for everyone. Yet capitalism appeared to be further expanding, with warnings (in late 2019) that a Trans-Atlantic US-

UK trade deal would end Britain's voluntary pricing scheme that caps the total bill the NHS has to pay for medicines. The US-UK deal could increase the NHS annual drugs bill from £18 billion to an estimated £45 billion.[40] For example, a course of sofosbuvir (a drug currently used to treat hepatitis C) costs around $5 to make but the current list price in the US is $18,610.[41] A phial of insulin, one month's supply, costs about $5 to produce. It is free on the UK's NHS but is sold in the US on average for up to $540. People with Type I diabetes who cannot afford insulin are dying from ketoacidosis and other serious complications.[42] A leading UK economist said: 'I can't think of anything more important than understanding what drives the inequalities we see today and working out what we might do to influence them.'[43] He added that inequalities affect every aspect of life. Yet his report records years of evidence-based policy papers and recommendations that have been ignored, with zero effects, alongside years of steeply rising inequalities. Why is so much time and funding spent on research and reviews that have so few real long-term effects?

Most research is not published,[44] and almost all published recommendations are not implemented. Even if they are put into practice, many practical reforms are designed, developed and tested but then fail for lack of continuing support. Despite numerous weight control programmes, the World Obesity Forum expects one-third of everyone in the world to be obese by 2025.[45] How might multidisciplinary teams forge stronger links between their different kinds of expertise and between their ideas (epistemology) and the lasting practical outcomes (ontology) they hope for? Health policymaking, and actual implementation, involve a range of disciplines, and CR theories can help to strengthen interdisciplinary work, as the next section reviews.

Critical Realist theories about interdisciplinarity

The COVID-19 pandemic showed how health and illness relate to every aspect of our individual and social lives. It highlighted the need for informed effective policies, from many relevant natural and social sciences and humanities. Beyond multidisciplinary grouping, it required more equal, integrated interdisciplinary work.[46] Debates about early responses to the pandemic included these needs on the four planes of social being:

1. all possible actions to prevent and reduce cross-infection; care of the sick, dying, hungry and homeless;
2. neighbourly and professional support for all in need;

3. government policies to maintain, as far as possible, the national economy, industries, services and amenities, with support for everyone in extra need because of the pandemic and
4. help for individuals coping with isolation, fear and despair and reliance on everyone's altruism and goodwill.

Each interacting plane needs to be understood in relation to the others. Expert scientific, political and ethical knowledge combines with analysis of uncertainties, possibilities, international examples, direct practical experience and moral judgements. This challenges the tradition that separates each bounded academic discipline into its own unique incommensurable grammar.[47] It involves naturalism that respects specific theories and methods in each discipline and resolves assumed splits and contradictions between them (Chapter 2).[48] When knowledge in every discipline is seen as transitive, and separate from the independent intransitive ontology-reality that is studied, positivist and interpretivist paradigms can both be respected. So too can each discipline's unique insights, theories, methods and potential for continual discovery be respected at the interacting levels of the empirical, actual and real.[49] Reality is understood as layered, not lying on the single actual level (flat actualism) that seems to support covering law predictions.

Scientists have to consider how their predictions, which assume fixed conditions in closed systems, are transfactual and work through numerous interacting forces within open systems – or do not work or are latent. Understanding the impact of COVID-19 on individuals, or on a village, city, country or the world, involves relating its effects to each natural and social context. Individual cases can provide valuable knowledge about these complexities, since each one is a concrete universal. It is both unique and shares properties with every other comparable example. All universals have concrete or material versions.[50]

Overcoming barriers to interdisciplinarity

There are serious barriers to coordinated interdisciplinarity. Non-integrated multidisciplinary teams tend to ignore how:

- members' basic beliefs about research (their assumed tacit metatheories about what 'proper' scientists do) are in conflict;
- they assume their disciplines are incommensurable – they cannot adequately relate or connect, and paradigms, such as of positivism and interpretivism, are incompatible;

- there is then likely to be poor communication between team members and
- rivalries are reinforced when university departments and funding bodies foster single discipline and sub-disciplinary specialisation.

Multidisciplinarity, without some agreed unity, slips around on the surface of conflicting world views or paradigms, and beliefs about the nature and existence of truth and knowledge and how we can validate them. CR works to analyse and overcome these divisions and to expand common ground between disciplines. This begins by believing that all research occurs in the same real world that we assume in our everyday life. See Table 5.2.[51]

Table 5.2: Barriers to interdisciplinarity and connections

	Multidisciplinary barriers	**Interdisciplinary connections**
Metatheory	No common team philosophy	Common philosophy or metatheory
Theory	Disciplines are incommensurable or all reductionist	Integrate different kinds of knowledge Non-reductionism
Method	Assumed to be specific to each discipline	Specific to each level of analysis
Between individuals	Poor communication Hierarchy	Mutual understanding and respect
Administrative and funding support for:	Mono-discipline research departments and careers	Interdisciplinary research and careers

More detailed specific assumptions and splits, which CR works to resolve, are summarised in Table 5.3. This table is quite full of jargon but, as with medicine or psychology, each academic term names a vital and unique concept. They have been discussed in earlier chapters (also see glossary). Attempts at interdisciplinary research and policy fail if teams do not identify and work on these splits, which are assumed in many disciplines.

If the splits remain unresolved, health researchers continue to rely mainly on positivism to collect, measure, describe and analyse data, to predict, to reduce being into knowing and to avoid searching for unseen causal influences. They therefore miss the causal explanations, which have to be understood and challenged before problems can be

Table 5.3: Resolving splits between often assumed tacit theories

Multidisciplinary splits: theories assumed by some but not all health-related disciplines	Interdisciplinary connections: CR theories
Scientism: natural and social science research theories and methods are identical	Naturalism: unity though not uniformity of theories and methods
Reductionism: research subjects-objects in natural and social science are identical	Naturalism: unity though not uniformity of research subjects-objects
Behaviourism: observe people and animals as if they have no thoughts or feelings	Reflexivity: respect feeling-thinking beings
Empiricism, induction, deduction: rely only on evidence experienced or recounted through the five senses	Layered reality, retroduction, research unseen processes
Irrealism: deny reality Epistemic fallacy: reduce reality into thought	Realism: recognise independent ontology-reality, that is discovered not invented
Relativism: all ideas make sense only in specific contexts	Universal truths and rights exist
Eclecticism: superficially combine theories and methods but ignore contradictions between them	Interdisciplinarity: combine theories and methods in ways that respect and resolve their differences
Evidence base: policies flow from evidence	Policymaking also involves moral practical choices
Functionalism: improve functioning, cost-effectiveness	Also challenge and change unjust systems
Facts and values are separate and incompatible	Facts and values are integrated
Hierarchy: from physics downwards	Equality: all disciplines make unique contributions
All disciplines are incommensurable	All disciplines can be coordinated
Gold standard: RCTs	Gold standard: the most useful relevant method

solved through real lasting change. They thereby tacitly support present unjust policies and distributions of power and control over resources and decisions.

Interdisciplinary research and reviews are conducted by individuals or single discipline or multidisciplinary teams. They consider a range of related disciplines, through direct knowledge and/or through literature reviews. Bhaskar and Danermark recognised disabled people's physical embodiment, their social and relational situatedness, their cultural constructions and subjective identities. They considered that researchers need some understanding of sociology, biology and psychology to understand any particular experience of disability. Researchers need not be an expert in all three areas but should examine:

> the possible contribution of causal mechanisms in other research domains, and draw on concepts and knowledge from these areas. [Disciplines cover] different aspects of the real, many have the same object of study although they address it at different levels and in different ways, and this provides the basis for methodological pluralism, but not epistemological eclecticism or methodological relativism [see Table 5.3].[52]

Complex subjects have been compared to a mountain, around which all the specialists sit. Each has a limited view, none can see the whole reality and all depend on combining their interdisciplinary insights.[53] Health and illness research (like global heating) pose extra challenges because they especially integrate natural and social structures.[54] Another challenge is that all researchers are affected by social and cultural structures and relations. They have feelings and memories and possibly fears of being ill themselves, and will perhaps subconsciously think 'As if it's me'. Physics is less likely to involve this personal subjectivity. A third challenge is time. Glacial melting lasts over millennia, whereas social responses such as during a pandemic constantly change in time and place. These challenges highlight the need for health researchers in different disciplines to think together across natural/social boundaries and not be constrained or divided by them.

Danermark has added five useful steps in interdisciplinary research:

1. initial planning phase;
2. disciplinary phase;
3. teamwork phase with cross-disciplinary understanding;
4. transdisciplinary, creative phase of epistemic emergence towards the integration of knowledge;
5. final holistic interdisciplinary understanding of the involved structures and mechanisms studied. If the research is to be useful, it must be disseminated in ways that return to reality, and move from epistemology to ontology.[55]

The need to overcome the splits and gaps

The next example shows how splits between the disciplines can be unhelpful. We researched the quality of care for babies in four inner-city neonatal intensive care units in Southern England during 2002–4.[56] We observed how the staff involved parents in providing practical care for the babies and in making decisions about their care. The four units differed widely in the clinical teams' attitudes and practices. Two were average, with humane caring staff trying to overcome institutional barriers between staff and families. In the unit that was least welcoming or supportive of parents, lead nurses set quite harsh rules and the medical staff were mainly interested in clinical research. The fourth unit was unusual in being 'baby-led'. Unlike the other brightly lit noisy units, it was quiet and softly lit.[57] The premature babies rested and relaxed in fabric nests that contained them comfortably like the wombs they had left too soon. Fabric nests were less common then, and many staff were not expert in fitting the fabric around the baby correctly, so that in other units the babies often sprawled in tense, uncontained uncomfortable positions.

I was then influenced by the social construction paradigm cited earlier: phenomena can be understood only within the context in which they are studied. To try to compare the four units would seem to break constructionist rules. I believed we should analyse and understand each unit independently, on its own terms, which were led by the views of each neonatal team. We were aware of the neonatologists' confidence in their positivist paradigm, their suspicion about sociology and their doubt that we could discover anything to report that they did not already know. I felt we should write papers that would present new sociological views, such as inventive analyses of time and space in the units. They were not impressed.

If I had known then about CR, I would have been confident to write about our views, which then seemed 'biased'. Instead of a vain attempt to be 'neutral', we should have been stronger advocates for baby-led care, showing its clinical, social, emotional and moral advantages, besides the serious problems it can prevent. In that light, we should have compared the ethos of the units, the many rules and practices that sustained each ethos, parents' views expressed in their interviews and the babies' responses we had recorded. We could have cited more of the medical literature on the health-giving benefits of encouraging parent-baby contact and baby-led care.[58] Yet this vital multilevel work is constrained by positivist methods of assessing and validating interventions. Each intervention is seen as no more than the sum of its parts, and each part should be evaluated separately as a closed system.[59] CR, however, appreciates that baby-led care, and perhaps all healthcare, can only work well if it is an integrated whole package of complementary, mutually reinforcing interventions, standards and relationships.

Jenneth Parker's CR work is useful in promoting the status of care alongside knowledge in informed moral agency. In interdisciplinary work on the climate crisis, which relates to healthcare, Parker argues that caring 'is the prime motivation for the increasing development of interdisciplinarity – but we also need interdisciplinary knowledge in order to help us to care more effectively'.[60] She cites a definition of care that applies to human and to ecological wellbeing. Care includes 'everything we do to maintain, continue and repair our "world" so that we can live in it as well as possible. That world includes our bodies, ourselves, and our environment, all of which we seek to weave in a complex, life-sustaining web.'[61]

Interdisciplinary commitments

Here are Porpora's sets of CR commitments recommended for interdisciplinary work. First on structure and agency:[62]

- Accept that the research subjects (people, institutions, services) actually and independently exist and are real.
- Scientifically examine patterns of events and aim to explain them by retroduction, by exploring the deeper reality of structures and mechanisms and transfactual theories.
- Use judgemental rationality to decide among competing theories.
- Be interpretive when examining the agents' beliefs and behaviours.
- Use transformational model of social activity and morphogenesis to see how agents experience structures, are enabled and constrained by them, and then react and reinforce or modify the structures.
- Work at different levels and scales from local to global, or at whichever levels are most relevant.

Summary

Changes to policies and practices have to occur at every level if they are to be real and lasting, as research on the interacting four planes of social being can both explain and analyse. The four planes are also useful for combining clinical and social, qualitative and quantitative interdisciplinary research. Small empirical studies may be nested within reviews of much larger political, economic or historical contexts in order to address large complex questions. Examples include the new epidemics of viral disease and of non-communicable (or lifestyle) diseases or the effects of austerity politics on health and wellbeing, studied in political-medical-social research,[63] or the impact of pollution on child health,[64] in which CR can be so useful.[65]

Previous chapters have reviewed dichotomies: positivism and interpretivism, structure and agency, facts and values. They have also begun to show how the dichotomies can be resolved and drawn together into interaction. The next chapter is about one of the most powerful concepts in CR, which resolves dichotomies and draws together all aspects of health and illness research. It works for transformative change over time: dialectical critical realism.

Questions to write or talk about with colleagues

1. Chose a type of person or group and go through the four planes of social being to show how health research can apply them.
2. Divide a page into four sections and note the parts of your research that fit into each of the four planes of social being.
3. List examples of enablers and barriers to mental or physical health on each of the four planes of social being.
4. How could the laminated system (Example 5.2) be helpful to your research?
5. How could CR interdisciplinarity theories inform your research?

6

Researching transformative change over time

> Jerome, aged 14, is in a school isolation cubicle again for three days after he kicked another student. He feels anxious, depressed and angry. Recently, his best friend was fatally stabbed. Jerome is on an 18-month-long waiting list for mental healthcare. He used to be in top sets, but is now in third or fourth ones, and has lost touch with his friends. His father is in prison. His mother does three cleaning jobs and once more has failed to get all the Universal Credit payments she is owed. So after school, he is usually alone in the cold damp flat. He misses the youth club, now closed, where he could be warm and relax with friends, have fun, play music, and talk to supportive adults. He has been to A&E twice with knife wounds and was told to go to his GP for follow-up care. But the receptionists did not see this as urgent enough and told him he would have to wait for three weeks, so he did not make an appointment.[1]

There were 4.1 million children living in poverty in the UK in 2017–18, 30 per cent of everyone aged under 18 years and up to 58 per cent in the most deprived areas.[2] How can critical realism (CR) add to the present extensive health and illness research about them? This chapter summarises a range of useful CR concepts linked to transformative change over time.

Research reports tend to be static, presenting data about a brief period in the lives of the people concerned. Even longitudinal research tends to collect moments or episodes at intervals during participants' lifetimes like a series of photos. And although multivariate analysis links earlier events to later ones (such as early years' experiences and later health levels),[3] there may be little sense of how or why these connect, apart from the timeless coincidence of correlation. Positivist researchers evade temporal analysis when they stay at the empirical and actual levels of evidence, discrete events and fixed effects but do not show the time sequences from unseen causes to evident effects. This chapter is about how research on processes of change can be more like a film, showing continuities, sequences and connections.

CR appreciates that open systems work in complex cause-effect chains. They apply to Jerome's multifactor descent into severe depression. In CR, everything is tensed (positioned in time), emerging from and then absenting into the geo-historical past, through many overlapping, converging and contradictory rhythms in transformational model of social activity (TMSA) and morphogenesis.[4] Agents are understood to be partly their continuing former selves and partly their new emerging selves interacting with social contexts. Events are rhythmic, in the varying fast or slow pace in cause-effect sequences.[5] Long-lasting problems in hospitals may suddenly be partly resolved. For decades there were long-stay tuberculosis and leprosy hospitals. When at last effective treatments were developed the healthcare was transformed, rapidly in some countries, slowly in others. Another CR concern with time is the critical tradition of looking to the future and hoping to change the world as well as to understand it (Chapters 4 and 7). All research that points out problems, randomised control trials for example, implies there could be a better future alternative. Yet positivist emphases on evidence examine past and current events but not future possibilities.

Dialectic involves the search for truth through dialogue. One of the most useful research concepts, dialectic is unfortunately not widely used or understood. Its critical morality interacts between concrete and abstract, structure and agency, facts and values. Dialectic can reflect on power2 oppression, need, want and desire. It is a guide and 'inner urge that flows universally from the logic of elemental absence' to absent those absences and work towards power1.[6] Some concepts that assist dialectical research will be considered first. These are: understanding absence as well as presence; difference versus transformative change; emergence, and immanent critique. Then the four stages of dialectical critical realism will be reviewed in benign, malign and mini versions, followed by an overview from past to future, local to global.

Critical realist concepts that assist dialectical research

Understanding absence as well as presence

Researching change over time involves polyvalence (many values). This is in contrast to the present dominant monovalence (single value), which attends only to the present and the evident. Attention to polyvalence, or the many values of presence and absence, was vetoed

2,500 years ago.[7] Like many law-givers, Parmenides (*c.* 515–460 BCE), confirmed by Plato (*c.* 428–348 BCE), wanted to preserve the present *status quo*. Parmenides vetoed talk of absence, negativity and what 'is not', saying we should speak only of 'what is'.[8] Bhaskar considered that the philosophers denied the possibility of real change by denying the polyvalence of presence-absence and of non-being as part of being. Like today's positivists, Parmenides saw reality in purely actual positive terms. Yet absence is central to presence. For example, to restore health involves absenting disease. The becoming of healing after long illness involves the partial begoing of the former patient's more dependent self and daily interactions with health carers.

Absence is at the heart of existence and the space-time-cause hub. There has to be empty space between words if a text is to make sense. Hospitals need empty beds if patients are to move in and out of their care. Openness as emptiness is essential for multiple possibilities and potential choices.[9] A world packed with presence cannot have movement or change.[10] Plato's veto on attending to absence has influenced science, philosophy and politics ever since. It can therefore be hard for us to think in these alternative forms of absence and polyvalence.

Yet presence and the present state amount to almost nothing when compared to what is absent: all that ever was, or ever will be, or is elsewhere; all potential; everything that never was and never will be. Absence is most powerful in that being and presence can only exist when there is non-being and absence. Absence can exist independently of presence, there could simply be nothing.[11] Absence is 'the simplest and most elemental concept of all'.[12] Absence and negativity are so immense that the positive is 'a tiny but important ripple on the surface of a sea of negativity'.[13] Learning, for example, involves correcting mistakes, filling in gaps and making so-far-missing connections. Absence and negation may be neutral or benign or hostile. CR is mainly concerned with resolving hostile absences of lack and need, from lack of food to missing thought or absent truth or logic.

Besides enabling and helping to make sense of the present, absence is a determining causal mechanism, a process like gravity. Unlike Sartre's vague nothingness,[14] absence in CR is structured by specific process and context. The infinite pull-push power of the vacuum absence constantly pulls us out of the past and into the future. Absence tends not to be seen as a cause, when it is assumed nothing can come of nothing.[15] However, Bhaskar cites the monsoon that did not occur,[16] so the crops fail, with the enormous potential effects of disease, dehydrated and dying humans and animals, violent conflict over scarce resources and migration. Another example is the longed-for baby who never arrives yet frames the would-be parents' daily lives. Many illnesses occur from lack of adequate hygiene or diet or vaccinations, and they are often unintended and accidental through lack of care. And healing involves the absenting of the absence of health or the negating of the negation of illness.[17] Natural necessity involves looking beyond the evident present in the empirical and actual and towards the seeming absence in the unseen unknown real. Absence is also central to the epistemic fallacy, when our actual ideas and perceptions are taken to be sufficient. The original referent or ontology becomes missing or absented. Monovalence can involve denying otherness and the difference between thought and being.

So to understand transformative change over time, we need to appreciate the polyvalence of absence and presence. In the early stages of research when researchers can feel daunted by their lack of knowledge and skills, it may be helpful for them to accept this initial absence as inevitable and real. It can be a catalyst to drive their work forward.

Difference versus transformative change

When Parmenides and Plato worked to maintain order and stability, they diverted attention away from the possibility of change by emphasising definition and difference instead.[18] An example is X and Y, or Y and X. Altering their positions makes a difference, but it does not change them. Difference is static whereas transformative change is dynamic. Earlier, Heraclitus (535–475 BCE) had seen change and flux in everything. Plato quoted Heraclitus as saying 'you cannot step into the same river twice'.[19] However, Alan Norrie's helpful *Dialectic and Difference* adds the more accurate translation: 'In the same river ever different waters flow … We step and do not step into the same rivers …'[20] Heraclitus's ambiguity allows that we and the waters are always changing but there is also continuity in 'the same river'. 'We' expresses our continuing selves, despite constant flux.

Questions about difference, change and continuity pervade healthcare over the life course. Some philosophers believe that as all the 50–70 trillion cells in each human body die and are replaced every seven years or so, continuity over our lifetime is not possible and we may become a different person several times over our life course.[21] However, CR dialectic combines transformative change with partial continuity within the same enduring though partly altered person. CR concepts (see earlier chapters) of being serious and theory-practice consistency connect our thinking about personhood to our own daily and lifelong experience of being a person with a lasting yet changing agency and identity (Chapter 3) and also of emergence, the topic of the next section.

Emergence

Emergence is a process and is therefore time-based. It involves one thing, property or system, which depends on and emerges from another thing, property or system. For example, consciousness emerges from mind, mind emerged from brain, and brain originally emerged from body. There is continuing interacting interdependence between them all; change in one entails change in the others (see Example 5.1). Reality is stratified (layered) as well as emergent.[22] Each later entity is more complex than the earlier ones. It cannot be reduced back into them or be explained by them. The whole conscious mind-brain-body person originally emerged from genes, but behaviours can only seldom and very partially be explained by genetics.[23] Decades ago, the hope that single gene conditions (closed systems) such as sickle-cell anaemia would provide a general pattern, and all physical and mental conditions might be explained by single genes, soon faded. Most genetic conditions result from multiple genes, and epigenetics explains how genes interact in open systems with environments to produce countless varied and emergent effects.[24]

Emergence occurs, and is a plausible basis for interdisciplinary analysis, in all the natural and social sciences. This helps to overcome scientism and reductionism and also seeming contradictions between the sciences. Body ↔ brain ↔ mind ↔ consciousness emergence connects physical, social and abstract entities within the coherent emergent systems and processes of each human person.

Immanent critique

CR dialectic unravels arguments through immanent critique, which unpicks and challenges the internal structure of arguments.[25] One example is Bhaskar's critique of the veto on absence mentioned earlier. The paradox is that Parmenides's warning, not to speak of 'the not', does exactly what he tried to ban.[26] Another example is Bhaskar's challenge of Thatcher's TINA view, There Is No Alternative to neoliberal ideology of cutting taxes and state services, such as the NHS, and deregulating markets in ways to favour the wealthiest groups. It is claimed this is enforced by international corporations and investors, who bankrupt countries that do not comply with their demands.[27] CR always searches alternatives, brings in new information, re-describes alternatives (see Example 1.1, Chapter 1) and unravels problems and contradictions by immanent critique. This can involve moving beyond assumed constraints at the actual and empirical levels to show how causal powers at the unseen real level can overcome them.[28]

Derrida's textual discourse analysis usefully reveals underlying binary oppositions, and so clarifies assumed ideas. For example, the nursing literature tends to confuse health promotion with health education, so that nurses' work on health promotion in clinical practice can remain unclear. A textual analysis informed by Derrida helps to unravel the related hidden assumptions that work as barriers to change.[29] However, Derrida claimed, 'there is nothing outside the text'.[30] CR refutes this irrealist epistemic fallacy and shows how discourse has to be about otology, its referent.[31] Following this review of ideas that support it, the next sections will be about dialectic.

Dialectical critical realism

The dialectical tradition of Socrates (470–399 BCE) searches for truth through critical dialogue. His student Aristotle (384–322 BCE) would examine a received view, then work through the aporiai or puzzles or problems that it raises, unravelling other people's arguments and inconsistencies, to arrive at 'a settled or balanced or consensus account of the view or topic'.[32] The three-stage dialectic (set out by Johann Fichte, 1762–1814) starts with thesis (identify the basic idea), followed by antithesis (negativity, contradiction, disagreement and conflict, critical challenge of new ideas and alternatives, discover basic principles and meanings in the first topic), closing with synthesis (reach a settled conclusion, a totality, new understanding by combining them into a higher level).

Hegel (1770–1831) saw history as progress that emerges from a series of contradictions through dialectic. Each new movement attempts to resolve contradictions in the preceding one. Understanding develops through difficulty and opposition, to be resolved by negating negations – overcoming problems. Marx (1819–83) and Engels (1820–95) developed Hegel's thought dialectic (epistemology) by centring it on materialism (ontology) and 'real individuals, their activity and the material conditions under which they live'.[33] They too saw history as a series of contradictions and challenges but in practical terms of humanity working together and with the natural physical world to produce food, shelter and other means of subsistence. Marx wrote that his dialectic method was the 'direct opposite' of the 'mighty thinker' Hegel's, and he criticised Hegel's 'mystifying'. Instead of Hegel's independent 'Idea', Marx said, 'the ideal is nothing else than the material world reflected by the human mind and translated into forms of thought'.[34]

Five tenets of Marx's materialism are also held in critical realism.[35]

a. The material world exists.
b. It exists independently of our consciousness.
c. Real though not total knowledge of the world is possible.
d. We are a (distinct) part of nature.[36]
e. The material world does not derive from human thought (idealism), but our thought derives from the material world (materialism-realism).

According to Marx, 'It is not consciousness that determines social being but social being that determines social consciousness.'[37] CR similarly analyses how we learn and know through direct, embodied, daily-life experience, common sense and theory-practice consistency. Marx believed, 'The question whether objective truth can be attributed to human thinking is not a question of theory but is a practical question. In practice man [*sic*] must prove the truth, i.e. the reality and power' and avoid 'thinking which is isolated from practice [in] a purely scholastic question'.[38] This is echoed in CR's epistemic fallacy, the semiotic triangle and *Enlightened Common Sense*.[39]

Marx's analysis changed the study of history from celebrating great men and their analytical ideas to researching the common people and their dialectical physical interactions with their environment in the struggle to survive and prosper. Marx's materialism differed from Enlightenment materialism (which still influences much health research) of mechanistic human behaviours shaped by powerful social structures (see Chapters 1–3). Many accept the materialism-realism of the natural world in the natural sciences. However, in the social sciences, many still reduce society and history into 'the ideas, beliefs and values in people's heads' to 'explain the nature of the economy, the social structure and the behaviour of governments'.[40]

The dialectic of absence and change differs from analytical philosophy, which influences most current research. The analytical ontology of presence and stasis (and 'evidence') normalises 'past changes and freedoms' but denigrates 'present and future ones'.[41] This is seen when so many practitioners and researchers resist major change.[42]

Earlier chapters considered dichotomies such as structure/agency and how, instead of separating them, CR examines constant changing interactions between them, in other words, dialectic. Table 6.1 lists the dichotomies that CR turns into dialectical pairs, different and distinct but inseparable and interacting. The dialectic resolves and transcends dichotomies so it can do justice to both sides in new ways. Each pair, such as positivism and interpretivism, are more fully understood and realised in their dialectical relationship. Instead of each being seen as self-sufficient, they are understood to be useful but incomplete, complementary and partly in contradiction. Like a river flowing through a landscape, or people flowing through a hospital, dialectic involves constant contradiction and opposition, which enable and constrain, reproduce and resist, reshape and are reshaped. The counterparts are 'apparently opposed but mutually complicit',[43] implicitly co-existing through their similarities as well as their differences. Like Marxism, dialectical critical realism moves beyond epistemology and reasoned argument (thinking) intended to resolve ignorance and illogic, by also emphasising ontology (being). The aims include overcoming illogic and errors and promoting transformative change and freedom.

Dialectic works in many ways, some of which are positioned in Table 6.1.

The emphasis on absence as well as presence, with Hegel's negating negations, can embrace transformative change in being and doing, in personal and political life. The three stages of traditional dialectic – identity (thesis), negativity (antithesis) and totality (synthesis) – are extended into four stages in CR dialectic: non-identity, negativity, totality and transformative praxis or practical change. The four stages are considered in the following sections.

Table 6.1: From dichotomy to dialectic

	Dichotomy	Dialectic
Macro	Positivism/interpretivism Nature/society Society/individual Material/theory Structure/agency Determinism/voluntarism	Critical naturalism, emergence, relationships, TMSA, structure as condition and outcome of embodied, conscious, social human agency
Micro	Body/mind Causes/reasons Facts/values Theory/practice	Emergence Reasons can be causes Ethical naturalism Enlightened common sense

Source: Adapted from Bhaskar, 2016: 44

Benign MELD

The acronym MELD stands for first Moment, second Edge, third Level and fourth Dimension. The four stages of the MELD dialectic are partly similar to the stages of a research project.[44] 1M, first moment, involves initial planning, questioning and the literature search, noticing sheer real difference. It is also like the anthropologists who newly arrive at the 'strange island', or at a hospital or community service. They stand back to observe unexpected activity and avoid imposing their own meanings or identities.[45] 'Non-identity' means that theory is not enough. The independent ontology must also be discovered. In each unique research site, researchers try to look below the surface to see the observed people on their own terms, making their own meanings and explaining their own lives. 2E, second edge, is an intervention stage, collecting data and making or observing or assessing interventions. 3L, third level, steps back again to take an overview of the larger contexts and meanings and totalities during data analysis and when writing the research reports or thesis. Stage 4, like the PhD viva, or discussions with policymakers and professionals on implementing the research, reflects on the whole process and brings new insights. The CR dialectic is cyclical and people return and restart at 1M with their higher levels of knowledge that open up new questions. The CR dialectic aims to negate ills and constraints on: human social and historical existence (ontology); questions of argument, reasoning, inconsistencies and contradictions (epistemology); and questions of human rights and freedom (ethics).[46] The four stages will be explained, followed by practical examples.

1M, first moment, non-identity

At 1M, 'non-identity' means that researchers try not to impose their own views or to identify, classify, explain or judge new observations by slotting them into the researcher's pre-set categories or prejudices. Standing back at 1M with 'willing suspension of disbelief' and 'negative capability',[47] which accept uncertainty, can open enquiry into deeper realities and new understandings. 1M raises the initial CR question: 'what must the word be like for x to occur?'[48] 'Any theory of knowledge presupposes an ontology [or] an account of what the world must be like for [that] knowledge … to be possible.'[49] What hidden structures, causal influences and patterns underlie the visible levels?

The questions can help to avoid a false, misleading ontology that could distort all later stages of MELD. Misleading examples include researchers who have been unaware of how their sexist or racist, colonialist or eugenic, assumptions inform, distort and weaken their research. False beliefs can become self-fulfilling prophecies and seeming validations and TINA assumptions, when misleading research findings confirm mistaken prejudices.

Plans for research about Jerome (see beginning of the chapter) would start from his perspective and those of his peers and the related adults to ask 'what is the world like?' for him to be in the isolation cubicle. They would frame questions about daily life in his school, home, local health services, community and nation, on all four planes of social being. Power2 needs to be examined in how it can diminish both the dominating and dominated groups involved (teacher/students, social benefit systems/claimants, healthcare staff/patients) and set up splits, repressions and alienation. An alienated person is absent, split off from the real, true, flourishing self they could be, the relationships they could have and the work they want to do.[50]

1M involves researchers' attempts not to over-identify or be intrusive but partly to detach or absent themselves from the subjects they observe. This is not through traditional attempts to be 'value-free' or to be a 'fly on the wall' supposedly unnoticed by the people being observed. Neither of these methods can wholly succeed, and they ignore rather than absent the researchers' inevitably influential values and interactions. These influences can then increase, unless researchers keep trying to be critically aware of them and their potential effects. 1M analysis leads on to 2E intervention.

2E, second edge, negation

Each MELD moment grows out of previous ones and drives on to the next one. Although 1M involves elements of becoming, these are central to 2E, second edge, process and turning point. Hegel's idea of negating negation involves change, the becoming of new events and states with the begoing or negating of former ones. At 2E, negating negations has three forms. Real negation is absence and nonbeing, which leads on to action. Transformative negation involves action, change and TMSA. Radical negation involves conscious self-emancipation and personal-political change.[51]

Again immense and almost infinite absence (noun) and absenting (verb) are central, if change into new forms is to occur. Real, determinate, causal absence brings out the world's dynamic processes and powers. Absence reveals and exists in aporai, which include omissions, ills, vulnerabilities, 'constraints, absences, oppressive power2 relations and inequities'.[52] These ills spur process in the need for transformation, in the passing away and absenting of ills and constraints, besides desire for what is so far absent, lacked or needed. Entities change but also continue without becoming something totally different.[53] Building on insights gained from 1M, at 2E researchers intervene (such as in action research) by conducting interviews and surveys and observing interventions by others.

MELD's concern with time includes tracing how TMSA, morphogenesis, causality, space and time all work in tensed, rhythmic processes that may cast shadows forward in long-term effects. Looking back to the past enlarges understanding of the present and future when attempting to negate negations. Absence also exists in contradictions because these are incomplete in their unresolved puzzles and problems, with potential and so-far-absent ways to remedy and resolve them.

1M generates developments at 2E and provides vital knowledge to inform 2E interventions. If researchers skip 1M and start by intervening at 2E, omissions and process errors may follow. Research with Jerome might start with the kicking event and see him as rightly punished and other students and staff rightly protected when he is in isolation. However, effective 2E interventions depend on 1M knowledge of what led up to the event, how and why. Research is also needed about whether isolation cubicles reduce (negate) the misbehaviour (negation) they are meant to punish or if they increase it. Jerome's other social, education and healthcare problems and needs and those of his family, school and peers would be assessed against interventions designed to promote young people's positive behaviour and wellbeing.

3L, third level, totality

The third and final stage of traditional dialectic is a closed synthesis. In CR, 3L is neither final nor closed, though it is a great synthesising, drawing together, of many aspects of life and thought, differences and dichotomies into totalities to understand their intra- and interconnections. Totality breaks 'with our ordinary notions of identity, causality, space and time' to see how these are not abstractions but are all interrelated. They are '*existentially constituted*, and permeated, *by their relations with others* … Intra-actively changing embedded ensembles [are] constituted by their geo-histories … and their contexts in open potentially disjointed process.'[54]

MELD totalities reveal present realities and future possibilities. Totality overcomes contradiction, incompleteness and alienation, as when abstract theories in philosophy are integrated into detailed social science research. There is the dialectic of unity-diversity, intrinsic-extrinsic, parts-whole and centre-periphery. Concrete means not abstract. The concrete singularity of each person combines their shared general humanity with their unique individuality. Ideas of collective wellbeing include each individual's interests within the parts and the whole totality. These can all be researched as human totality at 3L, drawing on detailed observation at 1M and experiences at 2E.

Research with Jerome could show how social and health inequalities and disadvantages work as powerful, pulling-down causes like gravity. Poverty and disadvantage are seen as real transfactual forces (that can work across both closed and open systems with different degrees of influence). Disadvantage may be countered by luck, or 'good genes', or support from families and friends and helpful agencies. Yet even if a fortunate few overcome social disadvantage and have successful careers, class and ethnic disadvantage still has constant negative power. This power over the great majority may be latent or realised, its effects may be visible or not and its influence total or partial. The disadvantages for Jerome include over-burdened, under-resourced education, health, housing, social and youth services and cycles of negative personal interactions.

Yet 3L totality is partial and changing, not final or complete. And each seeming whole or totality is one among many interacting ones. In the NHS, for instance, there is the totality of a bed space, the ward, department, hospital, local and national health service, all interrelating with global medical and nursing services and their changing knowledge, skills and histories. In the dialectic of events, each event emerges from previous ones. Jerome's physical and social isolation and distress emerged gradually through a series of losses, failures at school, exclusions and violent acts. All the events and interactions involve power, moral choices, potential gains or losses, with constant tensed becoming and begoing, absenting and negating. The interactions between individuals and social structures occur through space and time, in overlapping, converging and contradictory rhythmics. The totalities exist on all four planes of social being.

This practically infinite movement and variety could suggest the movement of stars in the universe. The stars have inspired the CR concept of constellations.[55] Totalities are locked into interacting positions and relations, such as the tier of health services just listed, in interdependent dialectical constellations. Smaller concerns are encased within seemingly opposite larger ones: epistemology within ontology, presence within absence. Change in one part changes the other parts. 3L shows how CR works towards resolution and synthesis in new totality but accepts that every totality is part of a greater whole. It is also mobile, open to change, reuse, reinterpretation and reintegration into new totalities. Everything is connected, 'constituted and permeated by their relations with others'.[56]

Problems addressed at 3L include splits and alienation and monovalence that deny change and absence, whereas polyvalence opens the way to potential and opportunities.[57] Research with Jerome would aim to connect many disparate factors and influences in order to understand and work with them more fully, with the aim of helping to connect him and his peers, teachers and family into more informed and supportive contexts, relationships and experiences. Effective mental healthcare would be part of holistic changes in his school, home and community, when everyone's health depends on their living in healthy communities and societies.

MELD looks to the past and future. Jerome is likely to be excluded from school, which can involve lifelong exclusions, with much higher chances of being unemployed and ending up in prison. The austerity cuts have ended most education and rehabilitation services in prisons, a false economy. Nearly two-thirds of ex-prisoners are rearrested, although that drops to under one-fifth of those who find employment.[58] This is harder to do for people with a prison record, or who are functionally illiterate, as half of UK prisoners are estimated to be. Many are homeless and are forced into illegal work in order to survive. Schools reflect and reinforce their society and political economy in the kinds of citizens they prepare their students to be, reviewed at 4D.

4D, fourth dimension, transformative ethical agency

4D continues the cycles of change through intentional, causal, transformative human agency and praxis (the practical application of knowledge) in personal and political change. These are essential in developing social freedom and justice, solidarity and trust. They all entail inner feelings as well as outer relationships and politics. Oppressive power2 relations can be ended only if people become aware that they are oppressed (or oppressive) and want to be free and believe they can make changes. Belief in transformative agency is expressed by conscious social human beings through their bodies, from personal behaviours to the political mass presence of street protests – about preserving the NHS for instance.

Sincerity and truth are central to the dialectic of political and personal change (Chapter 4).[59] Combined insights from both positivist and interpretivist, quantitative and qualitative research, structure and agency are needed, along with the study of visible and invisible entities, such as 'unconscious motivation, tacit skills and unintended consequences'.[60]

Poverty and disadvantage tend to be seen as abstract measures or levels, and interpretive research provides vital detailed analysis of their realities. MELD research helps to expand these personal interactions and responses (1M, 2E) by relating them to determining structures (3L) and inner being (4D). In CR, morality, human rights, justice, freedom and compassion are all seen to have an 'objective real property' and enduring existence (Chapter 4).[61] Their detailed meanings are contested and practised in many different ways. Yet their core underlying reality exists in human impulses to promote them (Chapter 3) through 'the first-person, action-guiding character of morality'.[62] They are experienced in the suffering caused by their absences and the benefits of their rewarding effects.

So health research about Jerome can neither be value-free nor add an external morality. Realistic research uncovers intrinsic morality and works to absent false, oppressive beliefs.[63] Schools with punitive 'zero-tolerance' discipline regimes limit students' and teachers' agency and moral choices. Teachers have to hand out punishments, which no one may question, and act as plaintiff, judge and jury. Students learn to accept anti-democratic injustices as passive witnesses or 'convicts'. MELD offers space to question these practices and consider healthier democratic alternatives.

Hannah Arendt and Zygmunt Bauman warned of the dangers of suppressing critical citizenship.[64] They identified three main groups in fascist regimes: the cruel oppressors, the majority of more or less passive compliers and observers, and the few brave protestors who act at great personal cost. Democracies depend on schools to nurture, not suppress, personal integrity and peaceful critical protest. Otherwise schools train young people to accept and even support injustice and to work for inhumane services, such as underfunded benefits systems,[65] or violent prisons.[66] Students need to learn how to promote democracy, restorative justice and conflict resolution.[67] These connect the personal and the political, and each person's past, present and future, towards achieving real positive change.

During the 2010s, knife crime in Glasgow, Scotland, was greatly reduced when it came to be treated as a public health matter. Punishments were replaced with support for troubled young people. This policy spans the political to the personal. Punishment only increases unbearable anxiety (which increases crime and illness).

Psychoanalysts work to contain and 'take in' their analysands' overwhelming feelings. Their method follows how, through their calm responses, parents psychologically 'contain' their babies' distress and thereby help the babies to cope with their unbearable feelings. They become later able to contain their own emotional needs, having experienced this reliable containment. If public health approaches to crime are to work, policymakers and the general public also have to change their own feelings. They need to move away from fear, anger, contempt and desire for retribution and revenge towards compassionately understanding themselves and others.[68]

Malign MELD

Benign MELD analyses problems and remedies through dialectic in the search for freedom and truth to prevent and reduce destructive cycles and resolve seemingly insoluble problems and fallacies.[69] However, malign MELD analysis fails to redress negative sequences and outcomes. Central to malign MELD is irrealism or the denial in abstract thought of physical, material and natural reality. This tolerates coercion, drives forward deceptive oppressive policies and leaves intact fallacies, errors, deceptions and oppressions on many levels, personal, interpersonal and structural.

One from countless examples is President Trump's policy to build a wall to keep out immigrants. The policy starts and ends at 2E, to negate negations. It ignores 1M investigations, 3L the larger overview and 4D inner reflection and change. When the wall policy fails, the only recourse is to try to repeat it. Malign MELD lacks transformative agency and promotes alienation and endism (vetoing any future change or hope).[70] This reduces powers to their exercise: power for its own sake, not for any positive end. It also confuses effect (the flow of migrants) with cause (the dangers the migrants are trying to escape).

Instead of insight, malign 1M falls into absence as vacant space, error and ignorance. The TINA complex at 1M (ignoring alternatives) 'readily generates' theory/practice inconsistency at 2E.[71] Concern with empirical and actual problems and failures to be negated overlooks deeper 1M understanding of causes, so that any reform at 2E will be superficial. Reports that attempt a larger view at 3L on the hoped-for achievements give few details of the complex processes needed for change. 2E interventions (build a wall) tend to increase inherent inconsistencies and contradictions, leading at 3L not to synthesis but to detotalisation and split. At 4D, inconsistent policies lead to lack of agency, divorced from intentions and insight.[72] Equivocation, duplicity, contradictions and aporiai (difficulty, want, loss, lack, need) follow. 'Underlying these are … the whole infra/super-structural complex from the dynamic of global commodification … to ideologies legitimatising existing power2 relations.' These are reinforced when human beings are trivialised at 1M and not seen as real people with needs and rights. Present and possible future changes and freedoms are then denied at 2E. At 3L, thought is disconnected and split through divide and rule xenophobic policies. At 4D agency is denied, with disempowerment and dis-emancipation of empty or fragmented selves. The central point of *Dialectic: The Pulse of Freedom*, with the importance of moral realism and truth, is that 'for a dialectical argument to be complete, it must show … the *falsity* it submits to immanent … critiques' and must join transformative philosophy and praxis.[73]

CR applies three (pre-CR) concepts that further reveal malign processes: veils and webs, reification and fetish. These will now be summarised. Veils and webs of illusion at the threshold of reality obscure and protect entities by keeping them intact. One such veil in Chapter 2 was the false claim that to protect hygiene in the Mexican neonatal intensive care units (NICUs) parents must be kept away. Immanent critique can analyse the claim as a veil in its internal construction and problems and reveal how it 'unwittingly expresses and presupposes the very content it would deny':[74] the policy actually increased cross-infection. The veil can be shown to mask and misrepresent power as if power is abstract, inhuman, apolitical, seemingly neutral and remote from social progress. That helps powerful groups to maintain unjust, inefficient systems. It also diverts attention away from examining the confused meanings of their power, whose interests it serves and 'the associated chains of errors, contractions and denials'.[75]

A connected move is to reify realities. This involves turning real people, processes and relationships into inanimate objects. In the Mexican NICUs, instead of promoting breastfeeding in active baby-mother relationships, the nurses reified this whole process and relationship into the milk. They sent mothers to the expressing room and kept babies and mothers apart, and the nurses tube-fed the babies with the expressed milk. All the processes perversely incurred very high infection risks and very low rates of actual breastfeeding.[76]

A further step was to make a fetish of the milk. All nursing attention centred on 2E, obtaining the 'golden fluid', though in ways that reduced distressed mothers' ability to provide it. A fetish is something alienated, suppressed and excluded, seemingly absent although it is central to explaining denials, inconsistencies and contradictions.[77] As a fetish, the milk was subconsciously associated with magical powers and was used to help staff cope with their fears by masking and mystifying deep anxieties and psychic wounds.[78] It helped to reduce their contact with anxious parents. At some level the staff knew their policies distressed families and contributed to the 25 per cent mortality rate. Yet concentrating on the milk seemed to enable them, at 4D, to reject and deny these painful insights and to claim they were doing all they could to resolve the problems they were increasing. Benign MELD follows process and progress; malign MELD reveals blocks and barriers.

Mini-MELD

MELD tends to be discussed on the larger scale of whole research or policy programmes. Yet just as natural necessity illuminates almost any topic, MELD ranges from macro to micro analyses. I suggest that clinical practice is a series of mini-MELDs, which highlight theory/practice consistencies. In each session with a patient, healthcare practitioners:

1M) hold back from jumping to conclusions and carefully assess each patient's changing condition;
2E) intervene by giving care and treatment;
3L) assess the effects in the larger concerns of the patient's wellbeing and those of their other patients, their colleagues, healthcare systems and budgets (such as whether to discharge a patient or not); and
4D) often reflect on their practice and how they and their service can gain from the experience and improve the care. They return to 1M in the next similar case, with new insights.

Practitioners provide healthcare through this benign thinking-acting MELD process of personal relationships. If they cannot exercise their autonomous competence through their chosen whole MELD cycle, they are dissatisfied and may feel very stressed.[79] For example, many nurses do not have the time to give adequate care to elderly patients at home when managers overfill their daily schedules.

The MELD cycle positions work on all four planes of human nature and social life, understood within national and global political contexts.[80] They show how intended benign MELD may be forced into a malign MELD. The critical realist and nurse Samuel Porter relates this kind of analysis of process to research and to 3L totality or matrix.

> Specific aspects of the social world connect with each other in a matrix of relationships so that no social form exists in isolation, sufficient unto itself. The consequence … for social scientists is that, depending on the question they are asking, they may need to look beyond the particular towards the matrix for their answer.[81]

The MELD framework can help researchers and practitioners become more aware of their autonomy as a process that connects past, present and future. MELD exposes how managers intervene to support or else undermine practitioners' professional autonomy.

To return to the example of the Mexican neonatal units,[82] they showed contradictions between: the needs of the babies and mothers and of the staff; the care some staff wished they could give versus actual care provided and routines enforced; the budgets and resources provided and those that were needed. A MELD analysis of each group's viewpoint, in relation to feeding the babies, could show the contradictions. Table 6.2 offers a basis for new planning.

Contradictions recorded in Table 6.2 could clarify basic problems. Progress has to be made at every level if it is not to fade away when related problems continue at unaltered levels. They include real causal levels of class and gender divisions, besides interpersonal relationships. The original campaigns in the 1970s to welcome parents into NICUs

Table 6.2: Feeding babies in NICU: differing perspectives

Group What they contribute, would like to contribute and what they receive	1M Needs, Resources, Constraints, Aims – hopes, Absences, Motives	2E Actual services provided or received, Interventions-activities, Negations	3L Staff-family relations, NICU design and routines, Barriers of racism, sexism, class	4D Hopes and plans for family-centred care and for reducing mortality rates, Personal-political change, rewards and risks
Managers				
Doctors				
Nurses				
Effects on babies				
Mothers				
Fathers				

were informed by research about how early separation in NICU seriously damages later mother-baby relationships.[83]

Example 6.1 applies multilevel MELD to research with children with allergies.

Example 6.1: MELD and improving care for children with allergies

Sophie Spitters, Imperial College London, UK

The aim of my doctoral research was to understand how child allergy health services can be improved locally. My secondary aim was to use these findings for practical recommendations for future improvements elsewhere. I studied four quality improvement (QI) teams who were improving their child allergy health services, implementing a previously successful integrated care intervention.[84] In my ethnographic study, I observed and interviewed team members and analysed documents. I discovered the CR framework MELD only after initial data analysis. Since then, I have used it to analyse transformational change, to critically review my initial analysis and to structure and strengthen my findings.

First moment (1M): non-identity

UK health services have not been meeting the needs of allergic children. There are insufficient specialist services and inadequately trained GPs and hospital doctors, and care is not well coordinated. A national review first highlighted these problems in 2003 with little progress since[85]. This problem formed the starting point for my study, framing its design and analysis. However, 1M helped me realise that I had judged the situation without truly understanding the *real* underlying issues and causes. Returning to the literature, I then (re-)explored the characteristics of allergic disease, the allergic child and the healthcare system to explain why UK allergy services are not meeting children's needs. For example, I found that physiological mechanisms underpinning allergic disease cause diverse symptoms affecting the airways, skin and digestive organs, with different disease expressions across individuals. As a result, allergies are often not recognised and treated holistically. Instead, respiratory doctors might treat allergic asthma and dermatologists allergic eczema without coordination between them. Poor care coordination is also linked to medical specialisation, which historically developed to manage the vast increase in medical knowledge – incomprehensible for individuals. However, multimorbidity (being affected by multiple diseases at the same time) has increased significantly. So, specialised health services now need to coordinate and integrate.

Second edge (2E): absences, becoming and begoing

At 2E, I returned to my problem definition, appreciating that the above problems can be conceptualised as absences. These absences, such as a lack of training or care coordination, motivated the QI teams to replicate a successfully piloted integrated care intervention locally. However, during data collection I observed that all QI teams adapted the intervention over time. Eventually, all the interventions were different. For example, to identify children with poorly controlled allergies, team 1 updated their emergency department asthma protocol, adding a section to identify children at risk for hospital (re)admission. Team 2 focused on schools, designing an audit form for welfare assistants to flag these children. Team 3 used specialist nurse reviews in the emergency department, and team 4 did not implement any mechanism. At 2E, I explored these observations by conceptualising the improvement projects as individual change journeys aiming to absent local problems (absences). This opened a more in-depth analysis of local circumstances and dynamics to find the likely causes explaining why QI teams adapted the intervention.

Third level (3L): totality

Although each improvement journey was unique, at 3L I explored what they had in common and how they were unified. I found that all teams functioned within a common '*allergy health service improvement system*' (a totality) of influencing factors, consisting of: clinical capacity, improvement capacity, professional networks and relationships, accountability mechanisms and competing priorities. All these factors are present and influential across sites, although expressed uniquely in each. The system formed the environment of influencing factors that teams had to navigate to make local improvements. Taking clinical capacity as an example, in site 1 hospital paediatricians worked largely in silos. Subsequently, the team focused on improving multidisciplinary team working and coordination of hospital services. Sites 2 and 3 both already had well-established respiratory and allergy hospital services. Site 2 then appointed a community asthma nurse in the hospital respiratory team to improve community services and community-hospital integration. Site 3 already had this post and extended it to include eczema management. Site 4 already had community respiratory and eczema services but limited allergy capacity in the hospital. A dietetic post was therefore freed up to manage simple food allergies.

Fourth dimension (4D): transformative praxis

At 4D I identified transferrable strategies the teams employed to exploit or manage their environment. For example, team 2 had a well-established respiratory service (clinical capacity) running the improvement project (professional networks and relationships). Asthma was their local health priority, with many paediatric asthma hospital admissions (competing priorities). New standards to improve asthma care had also just been published (accountability). Consequently, the team decided to adapt the original integrated care intervention by (initially) narrowing its scope from all allergic conditions to asthma alone. They did so strategically, to *exploit the strengths* of the local clinical services, to *adapt to local needs* and priorities and to *use the new policies to convince others* to engage with the improvement project. These three strategies can help any future team to navigate their unique environment and improve their local services.

Improving child allergy health services is more complex than simply implementing a previously successful intervention, which explains why the teams made intervention adaptations. MELD helped me to move beyond describing adaptations, into using them as a lens to understand the teams' improvement journeys. Exploring the underlying causes of allergy health service problems at 1M helped me to judge whether the adapted interventions were still relevant. Observing the improvement journeys at 2E highlighted local issues and motives explaining why teams were moved to adapt.

Conceptualising the improvement environment, with all its influencing factors as a totality, '*allergy health service improvement system*' facilitated generalised learning from unique improvement experiences. Exploring how teams navigated and exploited their own improvement environment at 4D helped me establish empirically grounded practical lessons for future improvement teams.

Summary: MELD from past to future, local to global

Health, inclusive policies and equalities of status and income are interdependent. Health promotion works through interventions with selected individuals but also at broader socio-economic and political levels, encompassed by MELD analysis from past to future, upstream to downstream, local to global. It takes the so-far absent future seriously and invests in preventive care. Although that can be expensive, the problems it can prevent or contain are immensely more costly, from high rates of imprisonment, to uncontrolled pandemics, to the effects of global warming on billions of people. Researching these past-future ties involves understanding absence, transformative change, emergence and the critical analysis of ideologies.

The final chapter will draw together the main themes of the book to show CR contributions and suggest ways forward for health and illness research.

Questions to write or talk about with colleagues

1. Divide a page into four and note the ideas and data in your research that fit into 1M, 2E, 3L or 4D.
2. Are there ways in which one or two stages of MELD could be particularly helpful to your research?
3. Are any of the following concepts useful to your research and if so how?
   Absence; transformative change; emergence; immanent critique; dialectic; veils and webs; reification; fetish
4. Can you trace a benign or malign or mini version of MELD in your research?
5. Would you like to rewrite Table 6.2 and use it as a plan to aid your data analysis?

7

The point is to change it: connecting research to policy and practice

The Democratic Republic of Congo (DRC) needs continued international help with its fragile health services that try to cope with TB, Malaria and HIV, as well as Lassa, Marburg, Dengue, Nipah and Mers, which could soon become major epidemics, intensified by global heating, global mobility and trade, and crowded cities. Epidemics could quickly spread around Africa and to Asia and Europe. Effective treatment of Ebola means that 'if you can get to people and treat them within four days of them becoming infected, mortality will only be about 10%. A few years ago, it was more like 80%'. Yet healthcare workers and researchers in DRC and West Africa face 'extreme violence and fear, with colleagues being killed. It is a staggering, astonishing story.'[1]

WHO (the World Health Organization) estimates that two billion people have no access to toilets or latrines, and more than 430,000 people die each year from diarrhoea. Millions more die or suffer from other avoidable conditions, including intestinal worm infections and diseases that cause blindness. From 2011 to 2018, 'WHO did battle with 1483 epidemics.'[2] These occurred mainly among Black and Asian people, many already suffering from other diseases. About one in every eight people in South Africa has HIV and two-thirds of them also have TB. When drug companies occasionally develop treatments for tropical diseases, they are likely to overcharge. There are 100,000 Black people with sickle-cell disease in the US, and millions more around the world. Two transformative new drugs to help them were recently approved, the first in 20 years.[3] Adakveo prevents episodes of nearly unbearable pain and Oxbryta prevents severe anaemia that can permanently damage the brain and other organs. Each costs around $100,000 a year per person, and must be taken for life. The 'black' blood cell diseases, sickle cell and Thalassaemia, are neglected by

> research funders, whereas research about the 'white' cells, cancer, is heavily funded. This is another example of the great need to transform or negate present racist global health research policies. However, that partly depends on a collective change of heart and personal values.

This final chapter considers challenges to health and illness research and then ways forward and research about the future. The chapter title is from Marx's aphorism, 'Philosophers have only interpreted the world in various ways, the point, however, is to change it'.[4]

Challenges to health and illness research

The above reports appeared just before the COVID-19 pandemic began. They reinforce the six points with which this book began: health and illness affect every interrelated aspect of all our lives; many causal influences are seen only in their effects; these are very varied and partly unpredictable; health is a process affected by daily life; health-related policies are practical and moral as well as scientific; they often fail. COVID-19 revealed our closely interrelated world. Illness in one continent may sweep across others. When the rich world neglects or exploits low-income countries, their disasters can rebound onto wealthy countries. Investments and research by wealthy countries, to benefit poorer ones, might also benefit and protect the donors. New global understanding that concentrates on these many large and small connections is essential if global problems of disease, violent conflict and climate heating are to be addressed seriously.

Yet so much public and private life is based on disconnections: racism and sexism, oppositions of class and creed, and loss of community and solidarity. Competition between countries, companies, services, universities and schools has some benefits but also great disadvantages. The once united NHS is split into rival sections, in a wasteful internal market.[5] During 2020, efforts to contain the pandemic in the UK were delayed when the government refused to work with the longstanding national network of public health services and instead spent billions of pounds on trying and failing to set up divisive new private services.[6] The main news outlets ignore the privatising of the NHS, which is reported in small alternative sources.[7] Split thinking is at the heart of government party politics, such as the separation from Europe. The education policy promotes 'powerful' STEM subjects (science, technology, engineering and maths) but downgrades the 'weak' arts, humanities, languages and social sciences.[8] Hard science is said to exist in arcane, bounded disciplines, each with their unique theorems, grammar and predictive power,[9] unlike all other disciplines that are realistic about open systems. Disputes between disciplines and subspecialties are divisive, and when social scientists disrespect one another, can they expect respect from anyone else? Disciplinary discord leaves the media, the public and policymakers bemused and unimpressed and many students confused or cynical when they are offered disconnected pick and mix sociology courses. Health sociologists are rarely invited to comment in the mass media or on advisory bodies. They were notably omitted from the official and independent SAGE, or Scientific Advisory Groups for Emergencies, in 2020 as noted earlier.

Ways forward: making connections and commitments

The public health professor David McCoy commented, 'We must better acknowledge the limitations of evidence-based policy and recognise the importance of expertise, experience and sound judgment.'[10] The COVID-19 pandemic showed the glaring gap between medical science and policymaking, which the social sciences can help to bridge. They would not determine policies but could aid more informed conscious policy choices, processes and potential outcomes. A public sociology urgently needs a coherent totality that, like the physical medicine paradigm, contains and coordinates its diversity.[11] Coordinated sociology courses would show, as this book has attempted to do:

- how all the subspecialties relate to one another, positioned within larger concepts of social science;
- how and why the paradigms differ;
- their respective strengths and limitations;
- coherent, critical, practical ways in which social science can analyse structure and agency, society and nature, macro and micro, theory, culture, values, truth and transformative change;
- agreed theories about the nature of society and knowledge and how knowledge is validated; and
- practical ways of connecting knowledge from the health and climate sciences into public opinion, policy and practice.

'Medicine is a social science, and politics is nothing else but medicine on a large scale', said Rudolf Virchos (1821–1902) 'the father of modern pathology and the founder of social medicine'.[12] John Urry called for sociology, not economics, to be the expert coordinating science for organising and interpreting all the relevant information on global heating.[13] His arguments could equally apply to health research. Individualistic economics, he considered, cannot advise on urgently needed social structural policy. However, instead of competing to be the leaders, sociologists might achieve more by being the connectors and coordinators and under-labourers, at the service of interdisciplinary research, especially in analysing hidden and assumed theories.[14]

There could be public debate, for example, on whether vaccine research should be based on public health or private profit.[15] How can policies be agreed on transferring trillions of dollars into public health, sanitation and clean water, nutritious food, sustainable housing and fair employment to promote human rights and health?[16]

Sociology is so wide-ranging, covering any social topic or method, this can be a weakness. It is too diverse to have a distinctive expert specialist 'voice'. Yet diversity and flexibility are also strengths in research into the huge range of interacting social concerns about health and illness. The founder of sociology, Alexis de Tocqueville, believed that 'In democratic countries, knowledge of how to combine is the mother of all other forms of knowledge; on its progress depends that of all the others'.[17] Natural scientists working on the climate crisis find the bridging work by social scientists between science and society is essential and needs to be increased.[18] This work shows ways to relate natural and medical science findings about health into people's everyday life, relationships, social structural contexts and personal values,[19] as well as to promote political and personal change towards more healthy and eco-friendly behaviours.

António Guterres, the UN Secretary General,[20] listed essential interdisciplinary work. 'Only by coming together will the world be able to face down the Covid-19 pandemic and its shattering consequences. We must ensure a sufficiently global and coordinated response to the pandemic, then build resilience for the future.' He stressed, first, the need to suppress transmission of the virus with 'aggressive and early testing and contact tracing, complemented by quarantines, treatment' and a range of safety measures. 'Such steps, despite the disruptions they cause, must be sustained until therapies and a vaccine emerge.' 'Second, tackle the devastating social and economic dimensions of the crisis' and support low-income countries to prevent resurgence of the pandemic. 'In our interconnected world, we are only as strong as the weakest health systems.' 'Third, [build] more inclusive and sustainable economies and societies that are more resilient' to disasters, as 'a moral imperative and a matter of enlightened self-interest'. This requires 'extraordinary measures': 'a colossal test which demands decisive, coordinated and innovative action from all, for all.' Extensive information, strategy and clear effective communication are all essential to public health, he said, to 'persuade people to change their behaviour'.

Detailed warnings have been ignored.[21] These predicted the great potential loss of life and the wasted trillions of dollars spent on dealing unprepared with pandemic catastrophes, compared with the far lower cost in billions of dollars of prior preventive measures of keeping stores of equipment and developing new vaccines, medicines and technologies. World leaders were warned to replace their repeated 'crisis and complacency with a doctrine of continuous prevention, protection and resilience'.[22] Yet unprepared for COVID-19, world leaders reacted in 'a cycle of panic and neglect'.[23]

WHO, like the UN, was set up during the aftermath of the Second World War amid international longing for peace and cooperation. Globalisation makes WHO more vital every year to coordinate global health, but WHO can only appeal and work for international cooperation and funding, not enforce them.[24] More countries are electing nationalist populist leaders who oppose international cooperation, and more research is needed about why disadvantaged majorities decide to vote, or are deceived into voting, for leaders who betray their interests.[25]

Might the pandemic, like the Second World War, awaken a global movement for renewed cooperation? In this hope, many plans were published in 2020. One by Common Wealth covers economies, trade, tax, mobility, rewilding and other major topics.[26] On 'Reimagining public health' it states: 'Public health is too often overlooked within economic and environmental policy design, but the climate emergency is acutely relevant to public health: as its impacts escalate, health outcomes are projected to worsen, widening existing inequalities.' There is concern that 'marginalised communities ... lack control over their own health and lived experience'. By transforming economies, we need to tackle 'avoidable and unfair structural inequalities which drive ill-health in the first instance'. Instead of channelling funds into the most expensive 'resource intensive healthcare systems', funds could be diverted to support low-risk, low-cost, highly effective public health and healthy living. 'Our aim must be not just to repair the harms of a sharp economic contraction caused by Covid-19, but also put in place the foundations for a new economy, one that is democratic, equitable, and sustainable by design.'

The UN Conference on Trade and Development, UNCTAD,[27] has criticised the unhealthy policies of austerity economics, 'free' markets, light government and debt as the main engines of growth. The massive rise in public and private debts constantly increases the great gap between the few lenders and the many borrowers. Oxfam called for an *Economic Rescue Plan for All* to meet the pandemic crisis.[28] At least $2.5 trillion were needed to tackle the pandemic, prevent global economic collapse and pay people in need direct with cash grants. The Plan would immediately suspend debt repayments of poor countries, and a one-off economic stimulus by the IMF would increase aid and raise taxes.

These recommendations involve rethinking, undoing and completely changing many dangerous routines. On climate, even if we keep to the Paris agreement promises, which (in mid-2020) we are not, global heating will rise by a catastrophic 3° or 4°.[29] On healthcare, with overuse of antibiotics, routinely added to animal feeds to prevent infection and promote growth, antibiotics will soon become ineffective. Surgery and chemotherapy will then be impossible,[30] and ten million deaths a year from antibiotic resistance are predicted. Meanwhile drug companies neglect research into new antibiotics as unprofitable,[31] advertising companies promote mass greed and waste,[32] and economists dream of infinite economic growth on a finite planet.[33] Among the many benefits of change towards less commercially driven societies is the likely decrease of stress, addictions, disease, malnutrition, carbon emissions and air pollution.[34]

Douglas Porpora proposed seven interacting critical realism (CR) commitments for all sociological research, which have been one basis for this book.[35] Each project should be committed to:

- the conscious intentional agency of the people concerned, their experiences, motives, views and interests;
- human relations and interactions with social structures including competition, power and inequality;
- intensive methods (ethnography, narrative, history and case studies);
- extensive or macro methods (surveys, trials);
- metatheory – be explicit regarding the underlying theories and assumptions about the nature of reality, existence, belief, proof and accuracy, knowledge, perspectives and methods;
- truth – accept that it exists and
- the inherent values in social facts – objectivity involves being fair, open and impartial, but not neutral or amoral.

Porpora advised less trust in explanations and predictors offered by extensive surveys and statistics. He advocated greater trust in intensive research methods, such as ethnographic case studies and histories, believing these can support valid causal explanations and generalisations about tendencies. Like anatomists, intensive researchers rely on examining complex individual cases, not on counting hundreds of simplified versions. I would add an eighth commitment, a main topic in this chapter:

- connecting valid practical research into policy and practice.

The general public provides funds, participants and volunteers for most health research.[36] Researchers could be more accountable to them, by using the resources effectively and researching questions for which the public needs to have answers. Yet much health and illness research is not original, or well-conducted, or even published.[37]

Health and illness research and the future

All research about problems implies or addresses future alternatives. So should we think more systematically about the future? It is usually dismissed as a research topic because it cannot count as evidence. Since the 1830s, researchers have debated whether sociology should be a positivist, value-free science or should draw on the humanities and imagination.[38] All human activity is future-orientated, and the founding fathers of sociology, Marx, Weber and Durkheim, were all concerned with where present trends might lead. 'Weber addressed social futurity implicitly through the concepts of rationality and progress, ethics and values, purposes and motives, options and choices.'[39]

Urry was influenced by the CR concern with absences, which include the future.[40] He envisaged possible, probable and preferable futures and four hypothetical future dystopias. One is catastrophic barbarism if present trends are not reversed. He advised that predictions should draw on research about diverse, detailed and interconnected multiple systems. The systems include social beliefs, values, behaviours, habits, costs and benefits, consumerism, law and policy, besides social and natural structures and institutions.

Although they are not critical realists, the next three utopian researchers offer useful ideas for CR research. Olin Wright advocated 'emancipatory social science' to research real practical utopias.[41] This questions why we want change, where we aim for and theories of transformation on how we might get there. Roberto Unger called for democratic, incremental reforms that are desirable, viable and achievable through shared, practical exploration.[42] We might be able to act differently and more collectively in the world and open up new utopian possibilities.

Ruth Levitas contended that utopian thinking points us towards expressing the desire for better ways of living and being.[43] We can ponder systemically and concretely about possible futures by imagining an entirely different society. Prefigurative practice means that our attempts to live out in this world the relationships and practices of an imagined better future might make that future more realisable. Levitas believed that a central, urgent task for sociology is to imagine utopian future wellbeing: 'the fact that our imaginings will fall short and will end in necessary failure does not excuse us from trying.'[44] Sociology can uniquely understand the matrix of social interactions with socially defined needs, wants and satisfactions. 'Human happiness demands that we find ways of engaging with one another that allow less fear, more genuine connection, more love [within] deeper and more satisfying human relationships.' We can attend to what we 'might become, rather than fixed [ascribed] identities … [with an] insistence on utopian ontology as processual and dynamic'. 'Speculative sociology [which is] explicitly normative [is] desperately needed.'

The utopian method 'is not prediction or prescription, or even prophecy'. It 'must now entail multiple, provisional and reflexive accounts of how we might live' through imaginative possibilities.[45] Rather than blueprints (epistemology) the methods involve radical being and doing (ontology) through journeys that reach new horizons and understanding. The Marxist geographer David Harvey envisaged each local community working out its own way of living, through practice and not through top-down central direction.[46] There is constant, creative, critical, dissent, change and experiment, and it is about the journey over the arrival, though with an agreed goal (equality or better health). Each new horizon reached gives new perspectives and potential routes forward.

Radha D'Souza analysed flaws in conventional sociology that prevent analysis of social change and utopias. She then showed how CR totality can overcome the flaws, by containing diverse, contradictory contexts and structures, actors and values.

> A fact or event is the convergence of multiple facets of reality each with its own history and geography, trajectories and processes that come together at a given moment [in] the convergence of multiple domains of reality at empirical, structural and ontological levels.[47]

D'Souza contends that present sociology is too dominated by expanding 'the merchant's world view into the [whole] human world view'.[48]

Facts and events are atomised, and nothing counts as relevant except the specific transaction (like President Trump's deals). Sociological facts (and multivariate analysis) can be like abstracted figures in merchants' ledgers, extracted from their social context. Then only the fact is seen as authentic; events seem arbitrary and accidental; values, justice, absences and alternatives are extraneous or simply dubious assumptions. And these assumptions are taken to 'reify the already entrenched merchantile ontology and the forgetting of history and place, time and space'. This undermines attention to '*how* we can engage with social justice and global governance for a better future' and to the necessary preconditions for very different utopias and political economies.[49]

Three CR concepts assist utopian thinking:

1. *Ontological realism* is vital if we are to accept intransitive problems and remedies such as health and illness or global heating.
2. *Epistemological relativism* accepts that our understanding is limited, fallible, partial, socially produced and transitive. Yet real, independent ontology cannot be collapsed into fallible human perceptions.
3. *Judgemental rationalism* recognises our ability to adjudicate between ontology, epistemology and morality in order to criticise the present and progress towards new futures.

In CR terms, utopia is the eudaimonic society.[50] This is 'association in which the free development of each is a condition for the free development of all'.[51] Transcendental realism connects the ideal (abstract utopia that transcends reality) to the reality (concrete utopia). CR's grounding in material and social realism counters allegations that CR's utopian thinking is mere fantasy. Imagined alternative kinds of living and of resources can inform hope and counterbalance the limits of flat actualism.[52] Bhaskar argued that most people usually behave in trusting, generous utopian ways, realising their true self. And societies exist through default values of peace and justice, so that errors and failings are defined by their falling away from the good.[53] Lies only exist within larger truths, illness interrupts health and war interrupts peace. CR aims for 'a normative order informed by the values of trust, solidarity, sensitivity to suffering, nurturing and care in universal reciprocally recognised rights, freedoms and duties'.[54]

Many researchers could say they are concerned with the future in their modelling and other predictions. There are difficulties with the usual approach. Economic and behavioural science modellers tend to assume misleading concepts of human nature as selfish individualism.[55] Their over-precise covering law predictions are unreliable; most economists did not forecast the 2008 financial crash. They rely on efforts to standardise, to control (RCTs) and to predict ahistorically (longitudinal birth cohort researchers assume later generations will behave as earlier ones did). They assume that closed-system, single-discipline analysis works in the social world. CR researchers and utopians, however, address uncertainties, unpredictable human agency, tendencies and complex open systems. MELD offers maps for researching the practical, thinking-acting, incremental, step-by-step change that utopians advocate.[56] Each new MELD stage brings new insights and challenges, reviews and restarts that give grounds for hope of human progress.[57]

The academic splits noted earlier deny the origins of the term 'sociology' in notions of friendship. Sociology could help to build trust between the academic disciplines by developing with them the possibility of naturalism and ways to encourage governments to trust their citizens as responsible and ethical, working with them to rebuild post-pandemic societies. Chapters 5 and 6 looked at layers and levels through which lasting change occurs. The prosperous classes in nineteenth-century Britain disregarded regular outbreaks of cholera in the poorest areas until they themselves felt seriously threatened. Then they introduced public health and sanitation for all. Mike Davis,[58] author of *Planet of Slums*, discussed twenty-first-century worldwide dangers spreading from low-income countries to richer ones. But he warned that we lack the international solidarity required for real global change, such as the massive support needed by African countries. Unchecked, the dangers will destroy current international health, trade and politics, though desperation during the COVID-19 pandemic has presented new crises and opportunities for change.

Example 7.1 shows healthcare working at multiple emergent and interacting levels of reality.

Example 7.1: Contested understandings of mental distress in the context of neoliberal reform of community mental health services in England[59]

Rich Moth, Liverpool Hope University, UK

NHS mental health services in England have been subject to extensive policy reform over the last three decades. This has led to service transformations informed by neoliberal ideology that include an extended role for markets and targets, the promotion of user self-help and, more recently, funding cuts. My ethnography explored the implications of these reforms for how practitioners and service users think and talk about mental distress within one mainstay of provision:[60] the community mental health team (CMHT).

It has long been recognised that psychiatrists, mental health nurses, occupational therapists and social workers, as well as service users and informal carers, understand mental distress in different ways. The explanatory frameworks they use to understand, define and respond to such lived experiences include biomedical, but also psychological, social, and other, perspectives.[61] The particular frameworks used by mental health professionals usually reflect their occupational training and disciplinary knowledge bases.[62] Furthermore, differences between the implicit models of mental distress/illness in use can generate conflicts, which negatively affect decision-making and practice.[63]

Yet although each occupational group tends to adopt profession-specific conventions for understanding mental distress, my study found that in practice orientations were often more fluid and diverse. Practitioners adopted and moved between a range of models and perspectives, influenced by the context of their work. I sought to understand the causal processes that shaped these shifting orientations. By combining critical realism and reflexive ethnographic method, I developed a contextually situated understanding of the dynamic relationships between concepts, agents and the contexts of action.

I found two critical realist theories to be particularly helpful. The first is Archer's critique of a determinist tendency in some sociological approaches. This regards structural and cultural influences as exerting a direct 'hydraulic' pressure on the thinking and action of agents.[64] Archer, and critical realists more generally, argue instead that while a particular structural process may condition forms of social action, these are mediated both by other structural influences and agents' reflexive deliberations. Health service organisational demands, policy regimes and professional training and education may all exert an influence on mental health practitioners' actions but do not determine them. For instance, as a result of their professional knowledge base,[65] social workers tend to foreground social approaches for understanding and responding to service users' mental distress. However, in addition to this knowledge base, there exist other policy and organisational structures shaping social workers' practice (and that of other professions) such as austerity measures and the nature of the NHS as a biomedically dominated institution. Austerity-related resource constraints make it harder for workers to find enough time to meet their clients' needs while, in NHS mental health services, individualised biomedical interventions such as medication are often prioritised over social approaches that engage service users' wider family and community networks. Moreover these latter two structural processes can be mutually reinforcing: in the context of reduced resources, service responses that focus on medication rather than social support and therapies are less time and labour intensive and, therefore, cheaper. Each practitioner reflexively navigates these competing and conflicting institutional structures that enable and/or constrain their thinking and actions, choosing within certain limits how to carry out their professional role. This produces a variety of outcomes: sometimes social workers resist biomedicalisation of their practice and struggle to implement social approaches; in other instances they reluctantly accommodate to biomedical interventions.[66]

This example highlights the second CR theory, that society works at multiple emergent and interacting levels of reality.[67] In my study, I identified causal mechanisms along the scale from political economy at the macro level, occupational and organisational processes (such as those noted above or the increasing influence of service users) at the meso level, to the micro level of personal interactions. Moreover, I found that longstanding modalities of knowledge and service provision were also affecting contemporary practice. This illustrates CR's theory of social structures as dependent on not only the current activities of agents but also past human actions and beliefs.[68] While current organisational structures are primarily shaped by neoliberal policy reforms, mental health work is like a 'pentimento',[69] insofar as aspects of earlier policy regimes and their associated institutional features endure through sedimentation into forms of knowledge, practice and routines. These earlier regimes include the custodial asylum of the nineteenth century, the biomedical hospital system emerging in the early twentieth century and Keynesian community care in the mid-twentieth century. Practitioners continue to draw on the (conflicting) ideological positions associated with these regimes that co-exist in the present as alternative modes of thinking. Mental health practice should therefore be understood as a process that moves between these overlapping and co-existing levels of historically sedimented meaning.

This analytic framework, which draws attention to both spatial and temporal processes, enabled me to more satisfactorily describe and account for enablements to, and constraints on, the activity of individual and collective agents. I was therefore able to move beyond a deterministic and individualised account of how mental health professionals applied their knowledge and to develop a more dynamic and context-sensitive understanding of knowledge in use.

Summary

'Most major proposals for addressing or eliminating inequalities in health are located too far downstream to do more than address the immediate symptoms or effects of inequality, as opposed to tackling and eliminating the [upstream] root causes.'[70] The proposals thus overlook both past and future and so cannot adequately safeguard the long-term health interests of the next generations or lasting change. I hope the many examples of valuable research in this book, some by critical realists, much other work by researchers working with similar 'commonsense' ideas,[71] have demonstrated the need for explicit theories, concepts, frameworks and values in all health and illness research and how CR can help researchers to think about and work with them.

Questions to write or talk about with colleagues

1. How does or could your research inform policymaking or practice?
2. What kinds of changes do you hope your research might support?
3. Have you worked on interdisciplinary research and, if so, what were the main benefits? If there were problems, how might CR help to resolve them?
4. In what main ways has this book been helpful to your research?
5. Could the book have been more helpful to your research? If so please let the author know the details.

ABCD – Articles, books, commentary and dictionary-glossary

Articles

Among many articles cited in this book, Gorski, P. (2013) What is critical realism and why should you care? *Contemporary Sociology*, 42(5): 658–70 is a good introduction.

Also see the *Journal of Critical Realism*.

Books

Porpora, D. (2015) *Reconstructing Sociology*. Cambridge: Cambridge University Press is the most clear and detailed book for beginners.

Alderson, P. (2013) *Childhoods Real and Imagined: Volume 1: An Introduction to Critical Realism and Childhood Studies*. London: Routledge summarises problems in social science in Chapter 2 and basic concepts in critical realism in Chapter 3.

Archer, M. (2003) *Structure, Agency and the Internal Conversation*. Cambridge: Cambridge University Press.

Hartwig, M. (2007) *Dictionary of Critical Realism*. London: Routledge is an essential guide.

Roy Bhaskar's texts tend to be dense, and his interviews with two friends are perhaps best for beginners:

Bhaskar, R. (2017) *The Order of Natural Necessity: A Kind of Introduction to Critical Realism*, edited by Hawke, G. Amazon.

Bhaskar, R. (2016) *Enlightened Common Sense: The Philosophy of Critical Realism*, edited with a preface by Hartwig, M. London: Routledge.

Commentary

Healthcare PhDs that have applied critical realism include:

Mendizabal-Espinosa, R. (2017) A critical realist study of neonatal intensive care in Mexico. PhD thesis. London: University College London, http://discovery.ucl.ac.uk/1546182/.

Martin, K. (2019) A critical realist study of shared decision-making in young people's mental health inpatient units. PhD thesis. London: University College London, https://discovery.ucl.ac.uk/id/eprint/10071358/.

Green Hofer, S. (2020) Complexity, co-creation and social practices – re-constructing quality improvement: a case study in mental health. PhD thesis. London School of Hygiene and Tropical Medicine.

Online lectures:

Roy Bhaskar, for example,
https://www.youtube.com/watch?v=TO4FaaVy0Is; https://www.youtube.com/watch?v=8YGHZPg-19k
Philip Gorski and Tim Rutzou, for example,
Towards a process-orientated ontology https://www.youtube.com/watch?v=HOhyWg72eK0
What is CR? https://www.youtube.com/watch?v=U5TIyheQk7c
What is CR? https://www.youtube.com/watch?v=DCEktTDdBIM
https://www.youtube.com/watch?v=eeYi6TLGFMs&feature=youtube

Dictionary-glossary of critical realism terms

Hartwig, M.(2007) *Dictionary of Critical Realism*. London: Routledge is the best companion.
There is a glossary in Bhaskar, R. (2008) *Dialectic: The Pulse of Freedom*. London: Routledge.

Absence, as a noun and a verb central to dialectic; the force that absents absences and ills; the empty space that enables movement and change

Actual, evident and empirical, what actually occurs; **flat actualism**, reduces the world to the evident and empirical and denies the underlying reality of which it is the effects

Causal mechanisms, often unseen forces, which are real in that they precede and generate effects

Closed systems, a single power or force works with predicable effects(see open systems)

Concrete, well-rounded, fit-for-purpose, material in contrast to abstract

Concrete↔universal singular, interactions between each entity's unique and shared universal properties

Constellations, interacting concepts, entities and totalities fixed together in relationship

Contradictions, constraints or conflicts, external or internal, that dialectic works to reveal and resolve in thought or action

Covering law, law-like universal conditions with predicted inevitable tendencies in closed systems (see demi-regs)

Culture, the third main concern, with agency and structure, in Archer's analysis

Demi-regs, relatively enduring tendencies and repetitions in open systems, when causal mechanisms can be identified though their effects are possible or probable but not inevitable as they would be in closed systems (see covering law)

Dialectic, search for truth through dialogue, interactions between different entities; in critical realism the process of absenting constraints, splits, absences and ills

Dialectical critical realism, four-stage MELD (see Chapters 6 and 7)

Emergence, a higher entity emerges from a lower one; they interact interdependently but are irreducible (see SEPM).

Empirical, process of sensing and interpreting direct experience through five senses

Endism, belief in the end of history and of change

Epistemic fallacy, collapses and absents things into thoughts, ontology into epistemology

Epistemology, thinking and understanding, distinct from ontology, within which epistemology exists.

Ethical naturalism, the social and practical always include the ethical

Eudaimonic society, where everyone can flourish, subject to the laws of nature

Fetish, a reified thing (see reification) with power and mystery that is alienated and suppressed through contradictions

Four planes of social being, four social levels of human life: bodies in material relations with nature; interpersonal relations; social structures; inner personal-political being

Functionalism, theory that whole society functions for the common good, however unequal it may be

Generative mechanisms, see causal mechanisms

Hegemony, driving leadership of dominant powers and beliefs

Hermeneutics, interactively construct and reconstruct meaning

Hermeticism, keep checking ideas for their truth, accuracy and sense

Immanent, integral, emerging from; **immanent critique**, criticise an argument by unpicking its inner structure

Interpretivism, paradigm theory of social research that attends to agents' interpretations of their empirical experiences rather than to the actual realities experienced

Intransitive, enduring ontology, actual events that occurred and cannot be altered (see transitive)

Irrealism, denial of realism, supports actualism, interpretivism and monovalence

Laminated, layered, complex, as opposed to flat concepts of reality

Materialism, biological and physical reality that underlies the social (see SEPM)

MELD, acronym for the four moments or levels: 1M first moment, non-identity; 2E second edge, negativity; 3L third level, totality; 4D, fourth dimension, inner being and transformative agency

Monovalence, single value, ignores absence to concentrate on evident presence (see polyvalence)

Moral realism, morality, values and rights seen as having universal, objective, real enduring properties

Morphogenesis, (morph – shape, genesis – origins), the origins, shaping and reshaping of society and human agency through agents' interaction with structures and culture (see TMSA)

Morphostasis, static or fixed effects of agency-structure interactions

Natural necessity, three levels of depth reality: empirical, actual and the causal real

Naturalism, accepts that methods of natural and social research can be unified and used partly interchangeably but are not uniform or identical in their methods or objects (as scientism and reductionism propose)

Negation, intervention to negate or absent ills

Non-identity, at 1M recognises our partial, limited understanding of identities and great differences between our transitive perceptions and the intransitive realities we observe

Ontology, real independent being and doing, discovered not invented

Open systems, two or more competing powers with varying, only partly predictable effects (see closed systems)

Paradigm, world view underlying theories and methods of social and natural sciences

Polyvalence, many values of presence and absence (see monovalence)

Positivism, paradigm theory of factual research methods that test, measure, compare and evaluate data

Power1, enabling, emancipating power, **power2**, coercive repressive power

Praxis, puts ideas into practice

Realism, accepts the existence of objects, beings, events, structures and causal powers, independent of human understanding of them, and that they are discovered not invented. *Critical realism* also regards morality and politics as real. *Realism or realist evaluation*, qualified versions of reality that differ from critical realism

Reductionism, applies natural science understanding of research methods and of the objects studied to all research (see scientism)

Reification, treats human relations and processes as if they are things

Retroduction, (also sometimes referred to as abduction and retroduction) inference that starts with observation then seeks the simplest, most likely explanation by trial and error; new discovery, invention or connection; leap of imagination towards unseen causal mechanisms

Scientism, regards natural science as the sole valid source of knowledge; applies natural science methods to all research (see reductionism)

Semiotic triangle, adds to the semiotic pair of the signified (concept) and the signifier (words, numbers, images), the third element of the original referent or independent reality

SEPM, synchronic emergent powers materialism, avoids dualism, reductionism and splits between philosophy and biology; recognises that consciousness and embodied human agency (powers materialism) constantly and concurrently (synchronic) emerge from the material brain and interact with it, but cannot be reduced into it (see emergence)

Structures, natural and social structures can be generative, explanatory, causal powers

Synchronic, (syn – with, together; chronic – time) at a specific or concurrent time, whereas **diachronic** is through and across time

Tendencies, effects of competing causal powers in open systems, only partly predictable (see demi-regs)

Tensed, sequences over time, central to analysis of process and transformative change that avoids fixed, static analyses

Theory-practice consistency, an aim in CR, to rely on the same practical and moral theories in research as in daily life, and avoid contradictions and inconsistencies

Thesis/antithesis, the first two stages of the traditional dialectic that moves towards **synthesis**; MELD replaces these three steps with four stages

Thrownness, Heidegger's concept of how we are thrown into pre-existing, often alienating, fast-moving social life

TINA, there is no alternative, a fallacy that CR critically analyses

TMSA, transformational model of social activity, individuals interact with society when they are socialised and they reproduce or transform society

Totality, the larger view, vital at MELD 3L, which draws totalities together to understand their intra- and interconnections

Transcendental idealism, Kant's view that data are not simply observed and collected, as Hume asserted, but are understood through our ideas, which are the conditions for the possibility of our knowing and verifying experience; this denies realism and transfers reality into abstract thought (see epistemic fallacy, transcendental realism)

Transcendental realism, recognises real independent ontology and also Kant's transcendental understanding of it (see transcendental idealism)

Transfactual, laws, powers and causal mechanisms work across both closed and open systems in the natural and social sciences and are only seen in the effects and tendencies they generate

Transformative change, dynamic process in contrast to fixed **difference**

Transitive, shifting perceptions of intransitive ontology (see intransitive)

Wicked problems, bio-social-economic problems that are complex and involve different perspectives

Notes

Introduction

1. https://www.gov.uk/government/groups/scientific-advisory-group-for-emergencies-sage-coronavirus-covid-19-response#scientific-evidence-supporting-the-government-response-to-covid-19.
2. Ford, 2020.
3. Huang et al, 2020.
4. Horton, 2020.
5. https://www.bbc.co.uk/news/uk-53433824.
6. Boseley, 2020a, 2020b.
7. Dattani, 2020.
8. Cochrane Collaboration, 2020; Campbell Collaboration, 2020.
9. Case and Deaton (2020) reviewed commercialised healthcare in the US, which is spreading into other countries. They concluded that, since the 1990s, capitalism aided by private medicine has led to opioid overdoses, alcoholism and suicide that by 2017 were claiming the lives of 158,000 Americans every year. Criticisms from public health researchers will be reported later.
10. Macleod et al, 2014; Farsides and Sparks, 2016.
11. Bhaskar, 2008 [1975], 1998 [1979], 1986.
12. Dummer, 2008.
13. Hartwig, 2007.
14. Locke, 1959: 14.
15. Midgley, 1996.
16. Porpora, 2015.
17. Porpora, 2015; Edwards et al, 2014b.
18. Among many examples, Saks and Allsop, 2019.
19. Bhaskar, 2010 [1994].
20. Bhaskar, 2016, 2017.
21. Besides the book, the *Journal of Critical Realism* is a valuable resource.
22. Pawson and Tilley, 1997.
23. Sayer, 2009, 2011.
24. Hyphens denote consistency or harmony and strokes denote dichotomies.
25. Alderson and Morrow, 2020.
26. Bhaskar, 2008: 160.
27. Bhaskar, 2008; Norrie, 2010; Hartwig, 2007.

Chapter 1: Rethinking theories

1. Snow, 2008.
2. Similar to retroduction and abduction.
3. Price, 2016.
4. Bashford and Levine, 2012.
5. For sexism, see Baker Miller, 1976. For colonialism, see Said, 1995.
6. George Eliot's fictional historical ethnography *Middlemarch* (1994 [1874]) set in 1829–32 details how the brilliant Dr Lydgate failed when he set scientific honesty before tactful support for his colleagues' and patients' traditional ideas about medicine.

7 Foucault, 1963.
8 https://www.un.org/development/desa/en/news/population/world-population-prospects-2017.html
9 UNFAO, 2019; Lang, 2020.
10 WOF, 2019.
11 World Food Programme, 2019.
12 Oxfam, 2020b.
13 Wilkinson and Pickett, 2009, 2015; Dorling, 2013; Marmot et al, 2020.
14 Pearce, 2007. Far from predictions made some years ago about the climate crisis and its effects being disproved, they are tending to be realised earlier than expected.
15 Ellis-Peterson, 2019.
16 https://www.londonair.org.uk records toxic gases; http://aqicn.org/city/london/ shows daily measures. The average was 43 on 3 November 2019.
17 See https://www.trendrr.net/8369/countries-with-most-water-shortage-maximum-world/#:~:text=One%20of%20the%20most%20water-scarce%20countries%20which%20are,extent%20go%20to%20the%20water%20crises%20prevailing%20there.
18 WHO, 2019a.
19 Gorski, 2013; Porpora, 2015.
20 Sutcliffe et al, 2018.
21 Rønnestad et al, 2018; Dermendzhiyska, 2020.
22 Repeated studies have found that patients can have such faith in placebo (dummy) medicine that it appears to reduce their pain and other ailments, for example, Zhang et al, 2008.
23 Hume, 1748.
24 Blalock, 1969.
25 Porpora, 2015: 36–7.
26 Catton et al, 2019: 8.
27 Porpora, 2015: 36–7; Corry et al, 2019 on positivism and nursing.
28 Ye et al, 2015.
29 Catton et al, 2019.
30 For example, Krieger, 1994.
31 Dorling, 2020; O'Hara, 2020; Ball and Head, 2020.
32 Anon, 5 March 2020, https://www.ucl.ac.uk/ioe/news/2020/mar/young-parents-more-likely-suffer-ill-health-later-life; summary of Sironi et al, 2020.
33 Murphy, 2017: 3.
34 Dean, 2013 [1991].
35 Shaxson, 2018.
36 Marmot et al, 2020; Toynbee and Walker, 2020.
37 Tilley, 2020; Conn and Lewis, 2020; Merson, 2020.
38 https://uk.Cochrane.org
39 https://campbellcollaboration.org/
40 Dixon-Woods, 2011; Gough et al, 2018.
41 Macleod et al, 2014.
42 Glasziou and Chalmers, 2009; Macleod et al, 2014; Goldacre, 2018.
43 Ioannidis, 2016. Yet the dismissal of so much research, largely reported through the systematic review system in the Cochrane and Campbell Collaborations, does raise questions about their review system and its fairness and accuracy.
44 Glasziou and Chalmers, 2009; Macleod et al, 2014; Ioannidis, 2016; Goldacre, 2018.

[45] Farsides and Sparks, 2016.
[46] See Rose and Rose, 2014, for neuroscience.
[47] Retraction Watch, 2019.
[48] Gough et al, 2018: 282.
[49] Edwards et al, 2014a: 321.
[50] Edwards et al, 2014a: 321; Greenhalgh, 2014.
[51] Gough et al, 2018.
[52] Clegg, 2005: 427.
[53] Scott et al, 2013; Schrecker and Bambra, 2015; Smith et al, 2016; Smith and Stewart, 2017; Smith and Anderson, 2018; Marmot et al, 2020.
[54] http://eppi.ioe.ac.uk.
[55] Bhaskar, 2017; Sayer, 2011; Lukes, 2005.
[56] For example, Knox, 2019.
[57] McDonnell, 2013.
[58] Fox, 2011.
[59] Deleuze and Guattari, 1994.
[60] Gaventa and Cornwall, 2008: 178.
[61] Wadley, 2015.
[62] Cornwell, 1984.
[63] Oakley, 1981.
[64] Blaxter, 2000.
[65] Bury, 2001.
[66] Frank, 1995.
[67] Beazley et al, 2009.
[68] Goffman, 1959, 1961; Gobo, 2011.
[69] See https://www.bmj.com/content/352/bmj.i563.
[70] Guba and Lincoln, 1992, 1989: 45, 17.
[71] Alderson, 2013: Chapter 2.
[72] Ramasesproject.org; Pawson, 2013; Greenhalgh et al, 2015; 20 standards for RE publications are set out in Wong et al, 2013.
[73] Porter, 2015a, 2015b; Edwards et al, 2014a, 2014b; Hinds and Dickson, in press.
[74] Pawson et al, 2005.
[75] Greenhalgh et al, 2015.
[76] Pawson et al, 2005.
[77] Pawson, 2006.
[78] Dalkin et al, 2015.
[79] Pawson and Tilley, 1997: 150–1.
[80] Pawson and Tilley, 1997: 150–1.
[81] Pawson and Tilley, 1997: 150–1.
[82] Pawson, 2013: 87.
[83] Pawson and Manzano-Santaella, 2012.
[84] Pawson and Tilley, 1997: 216–17.
[85] Pawson and Tilley, 1997: 216–17.
[86] Wong et al, 2013.
[87] Pawson and Tilley, 1997: 217.
[88] Dalkin et al, 2015 : 49.
[89] Wong et al, 2013.
[90] Wong et al, 2013.
[91] After the Greek oracle at Delphi; the method assumes that structured group judgements are more valid than individual judgements.

[92] Hinds and Dickson, in press.
[93] Greenhalgh et al, 2015.
[94] Porpora, 2015: 9.
[95] Porter, 2015a.
[96] Pawson and Tilley, 1997.
[97] Parsons, 1951.
[98] Dalkin et al, 2015.
[99] Greenhalgh et al, 2015.
[100] For example, Mogre et al, 2016.
[101] Pawson and Tilley, 1997: 64.
[102] Adhanom Ghebreyesus, T., Director-General, World Health Organization. 2018.
[103] Kim et al, 2018.
[104] Aicken et al, 2008.
[105] Pawson, 2013: 70.
[106] For RCTs see Porter et al, 2017a; for systematic reviews see Spacey et al, 2019; and for evaluations see Porter et al, 2017b.
[107] Porter, 2015b; Hinds and Dickson, in press.
[108] Hinds and Dickson, in press.
[109] Wong et al, 2013: 1001; Hinds and Dickson, in press.
[110] Wong et al, 2013
[111] Hinds and Dickson, in press.
[112] Bhaskar, 1998 [1979]: 9.
[113] Pawson, 2013: 62.
[114] Pawson and Tilley, 1997: 219.
[115] Hinds and Dickson, in press, citing Brannan et al, 2017.
[116] Hinds and Dickson, in press.
[117] Wong et al, 2013.
[118] Gough et al, 2018.
[119] For example, the London EPPI centre founded in 2004, which conducts synthesised systematic reviews, has always been funded by the Department of Health; Bartels (2015) is one of numerous examples of research about individuals not contexts.
[120] Pawson, 2006: 18.
[121] Porter, 2015b; Hinds and Dickson, in press.
[122] Pawson, 2013: 81.
[123] Sayer, 2011.
[124] Pawson and Tilley, 1997: 217.
[125] Porter, 2015. Porter and O'Halloran, 2012.
[126] Bhaskar, 2008.
[127] Pawson and Tilley, 1997: chapter 2.
[128] Pilnick and Dingwall, 2011.
[129] Hinds and Dickson, in press.
[130] Chouliaraki and Fairclough, 1999.
[131] 'Integrated' has changed away from the service being supposed to be integrated, with community care, social care and mental health wrapped around GP practices. Social care could not be integrated with mental health due to contractual restrictions. So there was largely interorganisational integration within the lead provider (community services) and some loose attachment to GP practices.
[132] Pawson and Tilley, 1997.
[133] Marchal et al, 2012.

[134] Chouliaraki and Fairclough, 1999.
[135] Glynos et al, 2015; Hughes, 2017.
[136] Chouliaraki and Fairclough, 1999.
[137] Williams, 2008: 1024.
[138] Kuhn, 2017 [1962], saw paradigms emerging within new scientific contexts, so that coordinating social research paradigms can involve working on disarray in current social, political and moral contexts.
[139] Rittel and Webber, 1973.
[140] Price, 2016.
[141] Pawson, 2013: 71.
[142] Kuhn, 2017 [1962].

Chapter 2: Basic critical realist concepts

[1] Barber, 1962: 555.
[2] Reported by CR colleagues and by hundreds of students who have attended the CR courses.
[3] Bhaskar, 2010 [1994].
[4] Following Kant, Bhaskar, 2016: 6; Silverman, 2017.
[5] Bhaskar, 2008: 36
[6] Mendizabal-Espinosa, 2017.
[7] Alan Taman's idea. Taman, personal communication.
[8] Bhaskar, 2016: 47.
[9] De Saussure, 1983 [1916].
[10] Bhaskar, 2008: 22–3, 2010 [1994]: 52–3.
[11] Bhaskar, 1986: 45–6.
[12] Bhaskar, 1998 [1979]: 27.
[13] Lawson, 1998: 151–2.
[14] Næss, 2019: 475.
[15] Lawson, 1998: 152.
[16] Porpora, 2015: 21.
[17] Bhaskar, 1998 [1979]: 123
[18] Bhaskar, 1998 [1979]: 123.
[19] Bhaskar, 2017: 48.
[20] Bhaskar, 1998 [1979].
[21] Not fully reported until 1628 by William Harvey.
[22] Bhaskar, 1998 [1979]; Porpora, 2015; https://understandingsociety.blogspot.com/2015/04/gorski-on-critical-realism.html
[23] Bhaskar, 1998 [1979]: 9–10.
[24] Bhaskar, 1998 [1979].
[25] Bhaskar, 1998 [1979].
[26] Bhaskar, 1998 [1979].
[27] Alderson et al, 2006a.
[28] Mendizabal-Espinosa, 2017; Mendizabal-Espinosa and Warren, 2019.
[29] Research-based practices, Als, 1999.
[30] Alderson, 2015.
[31] NIDCAP, 2020; Mendizabal-Espinosa, 2017; Roué et al, 2017.
[32] Pierrat et al, 2016.
[33] UNICEF, 2005: see their website ten standards for baby-friendly hospitals.
[34] See Chapter 1.

[35] Profit et al, 2010.
[36] Sadler et al, 2016.
[37] UN, 1948, and UN, 1989, Preambles.
[38] Wright, 2012.
[39] Bhaskar, 2017: 30, which summarises the process as DREI(C).
[40] Bhaskar, 2016: 55–6.
[41] Lukes, 2005, not influenced by CR.
[42] Rose, 1990.
[43] Foucault, 1963, 1977.
[44] Williams, 2020
[45] Morgan, 2007
[46] Wilkinson and Pickett, 2009.
[47] For biological grounds see Pettigrew and Davey Smith, 2012. For social grounds see Scambler, 2018; Formosa and Higgs, 2013.
[48] Bambra, 2016, see also, Schrecker and Bambra, 2015; Smith et al, 2016; Garthwaite, 2017; Garthwaite and Bambra, 2017; Bambra, 2019.
[49] https://hctadvisor.com, 2018.
[50] Brandenburg, 2019.
[51] Bambra, 2019, 2016: 137–82.
[52] McKeown, 1976; Polanyi, 1944; Bambra, 2016.
[53] Krieger, 2008.
[54] Bhaskar, 2016.
[55] Alderson, 1990.
[56] Nuremberg Code. 19481947.
[57] Seidler, 1986.
[58] Alderson, 1993; Agona, 2019. See also Alderson, 1999, 2012.
[59] Bhaskar, 2017: 48–9.
[60] For example, Winch, 1958; Guba and Lincoln, 1989: 45, 17; 1992.
[61] Porpora, 2015.
[62] Porpora, 2015.
[63] Bartley, 2017: 199, critiqued by Scambler, 2018: 177.
[64] Critiqued by Dorling and Thomas, 2009; Porpora, 2015; Scambler, 2018; Bambra, 2019.
[65] Benton, 1977, influenced by early CR.
[66] Benedict, 1989.
[67] Lukes, 2008.
[68] Bhaskar, 2008, 2010 [1994]; Mervyn Hartwig's Introduction in Bhaskar, 2010 [1994]; Norrie, 2010, Chapter 1.
[69] Benton, 1977.

Chapter 3: Structure and agency: making connections

[1] Teeple, 2019: vii.
[2] Teeple, 2019: viii–ix.
[3] Teeple, 2019: xiii; Dasgupta et al, 2018.
[4] Kruk et al, 2018.
[5] Felbab-Brown, 2019; Moynihan and Cassels, 2005.
[6] NRLS, 2019.
[7] Teeple, 2019: x.
[8] WHO, 2019b.

[9] Belluz, 2019.
[10] Penn and Kiddy, 2011.
[11] Parsons, 1951.
[12] Oliver, 2009; Ryan, 2019.
[13] Bourdieu, 1977.
[14] McCarraher, 2019.
[15] Purser, 2019.
[16] Žižek, 2014.
[17] Bourdieu, 1998.
[18] Mindfulness and Social Change Network, 2020.
[19] Layard, 2011.
[20] Davies, 2016.
[21] Davies, 2016: 6.
[22] Bentham, 1988.
[23] Foucault, 1963, 1977; Rose, 1990.
[24] Wilkinson and Pickett, 2009, 2018.
[25] Davies: 2016: 9, 273.
[26] Fisher, 2009.
[27] Becker, 2013.
[28] See Chapter 6.
[29] See Chapter 4.
[30] See Chapter 1.
[31] For example, Alderson et al, 2006a, 2006b.
[32] Butler, 2006; Fox, 2011.
[33] For birth see Neel et al, 2019, and for death Røen et al, 2018.
[34] Geertz, 1984: 515. For a history of analyses of the self, see Martin and Barresi, 2006.
[35] Deleuze and Guattari, 1994.
[36] Fox, 2011.
[37] Charmaz and Bryant, 2011: 293.
[38] Goffman, 1959, 1961.
[39] Gobo, 2011.
[40] Gobo, 2011.
[41] Goffman, 2014: 5.
[42] Glaser and Strauss, 1965, 1967; Charmaz and Bryant, 2019.
[43] Glaser and Strauss, 1965: Chapter 14.
[44] See Chapter 6 on change.
[45] Glaser and Strauss, 1967: 12.
[46] Charmaz and Bryant, 2011.
[47] See Chapter 6.
[48] Miller and Glassner, 2011.
[49] Schutz, 1967; Miller and Glassner, 2011.
[50] Silverman, 1997.
[51] Miller and Glassner, 2011: 132.
[52] Turner, 2008: 9–11.
[53] Personal communication.
[54] Wylie, 2019.
[55] Lynch, 1993.
[56] Garfinkel, 1984.
[57] Leiter, 1980.

[58] Gouldner, 1977: 390-5.
[59] See the example about parents' moral accounts in Chapter 2.
[60] Silverman, 2009: 138-45.
[61] See Chapter 4.
[62] Schutt, 2006.
[63] Drew et al, 2008.
[64] Lowe et al, 2015: 198.
[65] See Example 1.1, Chapter 1.
[66] Mol, 2003: 5.
[67] Law, 2009: 151–2; and see Porpora, 2015: 68–9 for critical discussion.
[68] Oswell, 2012: 264–70. For a critical realist response, see Alderson and Yoshida, 2016.
[69] Latour, 2007: 71.
[70] Place, 2000: 183.
[71] Bhaskar, 1998 [1979]; Archer, 2003; Sayer, 2011; Alderson, 2013: 84–5; Porpora, 2015.
[72] Porpora, 2015: 130.
[73] Oswell, 2012: 41.
[74] For example, Oswell, 2012, mainly considers disembodied aspects of healthcare: psychology experiments, behavioural problems, child development, Foucault's critique of bio-power and eugenics.
[75] Bhaskar, 2017: 6–13, based on Gary Hawke's interviews with Roy Bhaskar.
[76] Bhaskar, 2008, 2016.
[77] Archer, 1982, 1988.
[78] Wyatt, 2019.
[79] Archer, 1988.
[80] https://www.theguardian.com/cities/2019/dec/08/bhopals-tragedy-has-not-stopped-the-urban-disaster-still-claiming-lives-35-years-on
[81] Porpora, 1998: 339–55, 2007: 422–5; 2015: 96–128. Porpora's numbered order has been altered.
[82] Bourdieu, 1993.
[83] Giddens, 1979.
[84] Archer, 1995.
[85] Porpora, 2015: 110–11.
[86] Sewell, 1992.
[87] Archer, 1982, 1988, 1995, 1998, 2013.
[88] Harvey, 2005; Porpora, 2015: 96–128, and 98–101 on ANT and Bourdieu's versions of type 4.
[89] Archer, 2000, 2003.
[90] Archer, 2013.
[91] Archer, 2000.
[92] Loach and Obiols, 2016.
[93] RE is explained in Chapter 1.
[94] Pawson and Tilley, 1997: 66, see Point 1.4 in Chapter 1.
[95] Bhaskar, 1998 [1979]: 79.
[96] Porter, 2015b.
[97] Pawson, 2013: 70.
[98] Porter, 2015b.
[99] Porter, 2015b.
[100] Pawson and Tilley, 1997: 66.

[101] Porter, 2015b.
[102] Pawson and Tilley, 1997: 75.
[103] Porter, 2015b.
[104] Porter, 2015b. See also, Porter, 2015a, 2017; Pawson, 2013, 2016a, 2016b; and the detailed informative debate, https://staffprofiles.bournemouth.ac.uk/display/porters#publications
[105] Marx, 2000 [1852].
[106] Bhaskar, 2008: 76, 90.
[107] Bhaskar, 2008 [1975].
[108] Archer, 2000, 2003; Porpora, 2015.
[109] Bhaskar, 2008: 198, 2010 [1994]: 58.
[110] Bhaskar, 1998 [1979]: 81; Archer, 2000, 2003.
[111] Archer, 1982, 2000, 2003.
[112] Kirkpatrick et al, 2018. This study is funded by the National Institute for Health Research (NIHR) Programme Grant for Applied Research (PGfAR) (grant reference RP-PG-1210-12011. The views expressed are those of the author(s) and not necessarily those of the NIHR or the Department of Health and Social Care.
[113] For morphogenetic cycle see Archer, 1995.
[114] Swenson, 2016.
[115] Fonagy, 2001.
[116] Bhaskar, 2016: 12, 53, 66, 164, 194, 204–5, 208.
[117] Bhaskar, 2016: 66, Figure 3.5.
[118] Bhaskar, 1998 [1979]: 97–107; 2016: 14, 44, 49, 61, 160, 182, 194.
[119] Morgan, 2007.
[120] Archer, 2003.
[121] Manyukhina, 2018.
[122] Sutcliffe et al, 2018.
[123] Archer, 2003.
[124] Archer, 2000: 318.
[125] Hartwig, 2007: 73–4; Bhaskar, 2008;
[126] McDonnell, 2013.
[127] Oswell, 2012: 264–70.
[128] PhD supervisors Margaret Jones, Peter Larmer, Kath McPherson.
[129] Vincent and Wapshott, 2014.
[130] Aadal et al, 2013; Clark and Wall, 2003; Hayes et al, 2010; Janzen and Mugler, 2009; Jinks and Hope, 2000; Pryor, 2010; Pryor and Smith, 2002.
[131] Koç, 2012.
[132] Yin, 2014.
[133] Davenport, 2020 unpublished thesis: 238.
[134] Davenport, 2020 unpublished thesis: 3.
[135] Archer, 1995.
[136] Fonagy, 2001.

Chapter 4: Health and illness research: value-free or value-laden?

[1] CPAG, 2020.
[2] O'Hara, 2020, and see the critical epidemiologists in Chapter 1.
[3] Dorling, 2020, in O'Hara, 2020.
[4] NAO, 2020.

[5] APPG, 2019.
[6] Such as when coordinated by IPCC, 2018.
[7] Thanks to Alan Taman.
[8] Marteau, 2018; Professor Dame Theresa Marteau, https://www.phpc.cam.ac.uk/people/pcu-group/pcu-senior-academic-staff/theresa-marteau/.
[9] Durkheim, 1995 [1912]; Parsons, 1951.
[10] Parsons, 1951, Chapter 5.
[11] Gouldner, 1977.
[12] Weber, 1968.
[13] Hammersley, 1995.
[14] Lukes, 2008.
[15] Mead, 1928.
[16] Hewlett and Hewlett, 2008.
[17] Mire, 2020.
[18] Lukes, 2005.
[19] Bhaskar, 2008; Porpora, 2015; Sayer, 2011.
[20] Hume, 1739: 335.
[21] Hume, 1739: 335.
[22] 'Reason' is derived from the Latin 'ratio', 'ration' or 'calculate'.
[23] For example, Philippa Foot, Alasdair MacIntyre, May Midgley, Hilary Putnam, John Searle.
[24] Bhaskar, 1998 [1979]: 62.
[25] Nietzsche, cited in Bhaskar, 1986: 200.
[26] Lang, 2020.
[27] Sayer, 2011, 2019.
[28] Sayer, 2017: 31.
[29] Hammersley, 1995: 14.
[30] Sayer, 2011.
[31] A version of Kant's imperative, see later section on bioethics.
[32] Sayer, 2011: 248.
[33] Goodfield, 1981: 63.
[34] Keller, 1985: 38.
[35] Shipton et al, 2018.
[36] Goldacre, 2012.
[37] Bhumika et al, 2008; Davis and Abraham, 2013.
[38] Holmwood, 2014.
[39] Therborn, 2014.
[40] For example, David Attenborough in his BBC series on the planet and Michael Marmot et al, 2020.
[41] Marmot et al, 2020.
[42] Taman, 2020, report of the launch of the Marmot review.
[43] Rempel et al, 2019.
[44] Dorling, 2015.
[45] https://www.rcplondon.ac.uk/news/marmot-review-2020-government-must-go-further
[46] UN, 1966, Article 12.
[47] UN, 1948.
[48] UN, 1989 terms governments who have ratified it 'state parties' and lists their duties.
[49] UN, 1948: Article 25.1.

[50] Nuremberg Code, 1947.
[51] UN, 1989: Article 24.2.
[52] UN, 1989: Article 24, 2e.
[53] Roosevelt, 1999 [1958]: 190.
[54] *Holy Bible*, Book of Exodus.
[55] Woodiwiss, 2005.
[56] Paine, 2000 [1791].
[57] UDHR, 1948: Preamble; the first clause is also in UN, 1989: Preamble.
[58] Ken Loach's 2019 film, *Sorry We Missed You*, shows the modern slavery of enforced grinding work to try and fail to repay debts.
[59] Smallwood, 2015.
[60] Sayer, 2011.
[61] Valentini, 2017: 862.
[62] Macklin, 2003: 1419–20.
[63] *Independent*, 6 January 2020, https://www.independent.co.uk/news/health/nhs-violence-hospitals-health-safety-hse-assault-staff-a9272596.html
[64] UN, 1948, 1989 and the series of human rights conventions.
[65] Broad et al, 2006; Midgley, 1994, 2002; de Waal, 2013.
[66] Archer, 2000, 2003.
[67] Bloom, 2014; Gopnik, 2010.
[68] This is neither to support nor to deny animal rights but to set aside these complex debates that are not directly relevant to this book.
[69] Smith, 2010: 400, 435.
[70] Bhaskar, 2016: 170.
[71] Alderson, 1990, 1993.
[72] Adapted from Calnan and Rowe, 2008.
[73] Pauli, 2019.
[74] Sayer, 2009.
[75] Collier, 1994.
[76] Sen, 1999; Nussbaum, 2006.
[77] https://www.worldbank.org/en/topic/disability
[78] Oliver, 2009.
[79] Haben, 2019.
[80] BBC Radio 4. *No Triumph, No Tragedy*, 27 February 2019.
[81] Shakespeare, 2013.
[82] Shakespeare, 2010: 266–73.
[83] Shakespeare et al, 2017.
[84] Gearty, 2011.
[85] Sayer, 2009, 2011, with important critiques of Foucault and Habermas.
[86] Sayer, 2009: 782.
[87] Bhaskar and Danermark, 2006.
[88] Bhaskar and Danermark, 2006, online version no page numbers.
[89] See also Figure 5.1 in Chapter 5.
[90] See Chapter 5.
[91] Bhaskar, 2008.
[92] Charlie Gard Case, 2017.
[93] RCPCH, 2020.
[94] Sayer, 2011.
[95] Alderson and Morrow, 2020 is based on Ten Topics, lists of ethical questions to ask at each stage of research.

[96] Bhaskar, 2008; Sayer, 2011, 2017.
[97] Beauchamp and Childress, 2013 [1979].
[98] Pappworth, 1967.
[99] Yet if research was combined with treating patients, British doctors were advised they need not request consent to research (MRC, 1964). This advice was not withdrawn until the MRC Annual Report 1991–92.
[100] Beauchamp and Childress, 2013 [1979].
[101] Kant, 1964.
[102] Beauchamp and Childress, 2013 [1979].
[103] Ravitsky, 2020.
[104] Fox, 2008.
[105] The policy always to name 'research subjects' as 'participants' can be misleading and mask coercion. It was more concerned to promote ideas of friendly research that people would happily support than to promote their informed decision-making or to share power. 'Participatory' research and consultations can be tokenistic, as noted earlier, with people being under-informed or their views being misrepresented.
[106] Doshi, 2020.
[107] Smith, 2011.
[108] Bentham et al, 1987.
[109] Influenced by J Bentham and J. S. Mill.
[110] For rights, Alderson, 2016; for principles of freedom, Bhaskar, 2008; and for justice, Norrie, 2010.
[111] Pellegrino and Thomasma, 1994.
[112] MacIntyre, 2007 [1981].
[113] Plato, 2019.
[114] Sen, 1999; Nussbaum, 2006; Nussbaum, 1999, considers virtue ethics is influenced by deontology and utilitarianism.
[115] Bhaskar, 2008: 382.
[116] Hérbert and Rosen, 2019: 19.
[117] A more detailed review is in Alderson and Morrow, 2020, Chapter 6.
[118] A major influence was the Belmont Report by National Commission for the Protection of Human Subjects of Biomedical and Behavioral Research, 1979.
[119] BSA, 2003, followed by ESRC, 2005.
[120] Personal observation, having been involved with healthcare ethics committees since 1981.
[121] Doctors contribute far more to bioethics literature, journals and policy than social researchers do.
[122] GDPR, the Data Protection Act 2018, the UK's implementation of the European General Data Protection Regulation.
[123] Barnett et al, 2016; Clay-Williams et al, 2018.
[124] Shown on the NHS Health Research Authority site, www.hra.ac.uk
[125] Critics include: Shweder, 2006; White, 2007; Hedgecoe, 2016; Holmwood, 2010; Stanley and Wise, 2010; Dingwall, 2008, 2018; Hammersley and Traianou, 2014. A more detailed review is in Alderson and Morrow, 2020, Chapter 6.
[126] Dingwall, 2018: 17.
[127] Shweder, 2006: 514.
[128] Kleinman et al, 1997.
[129] De Vries and Henley, 2014: 85–6.
[130] Bhaskar, 2008: 281; Porpora, 2015: 142–3.
[131] Bhaskar, 2008; Lukes, 2008; Sayer, 2011.

[132] Fox, 2008; Holmwood, 2010; Lincoln, 1995: 277–8; Mertens et al, 2009: 88; Edwards and Mauthner, 2012.
[133] Denzin and Giardina, 2007: 12.
[134] Wassenaar and Mamotte, 2012: 274.
[135] Smith, 2005: 85–8; Metz, 2013; Israel, 2018.
[136] Morreira, 2012; Metz, 2013.
[137] Posel and Ross, 2014: 3.
[138] Alderson et al, 2020.
[139] Fox, 2008.
[140] Bhaskar, 1998 [1979]: 259–62; Archer, 2003; Sayer, 2011.
[141] Mendizabal-Espinosa, 2017; Mendizabal-Espinosa and Warren, 2019. See Chapter 2, Example 2.1. There was a similar challenge for Alderson et al, 2005.
[142] Sayer, 2000: 159.
[143] Bhaskar, 2016: 137.
[144] Bentham et al, 1987.
[145] Bartley, 2017: 199, 201.
[146] Porpora, 2015; Sayer, 2011; Scambler, 2018.
[147] Bambra et al, 2007: 572.
[148] Sayer, 2020.
[149] Schrecker and Bambra, 2015; Bambra, 2016, 2019; Smith et al, 2016; Garthwaite and Bambra, 2017; Smith and Stewart, 2017; Smith and Anderson, 2018.
[150] Wilkinson and Pickett, 2009, 2018.
[151] There Is No Alternative.
[152] Bourdieu, 1998.
[153] Harvey, 2005.
[154] Klein, 2007; Mirowski, 2014; Mirowski and Plehwe, 2009.
[155] Navarro, 2020.
[156] Schrecker and Bambra, 2015.
[157] Habermas, 1987; see also Planes of social being, in Chapter 5.
[158] INVOLVE, 2012.
[159] Bissell et al, 2019.
[160] See Chapters 1 and 3.
[161] Pawson, 2016a, 2016b; Porter, 2015a, 2015b, 2017.
[162] Pawson, 2013: 81; 2006: 18.
[163] Pawson and Tilley, 1997: 135.
[164] Porter, 2015b: 65; Hinds and Dickson, 2018.
[165] Pawson and Tilley, 1997: 217.
[166] See Chapter 3.
[167] Porter, 2015b: 76.
[168] Porter and O'Halloran, 2012.
[169] Popper, 1945 [2011]. Popper was a founder of neoliberalism (Mirowski and Plehwe, 2009: 21) and also inspired evidence-based medicine (Chalmers, 2005).
[170] Porter, 2015b: 77. For lifeworlds see Example 4.1.
[171] Tilley, 2020, discussed further in Chapter 7.
[172] Pawson, 2013:474.
[173] Porter, 2015b: 77.
[174] Gough et al, 2018: 284–7.
[175] DfE, 2019.
[176] Kurtz et al, 2005; Hall and Hall, 2007.
[177] CYPMHC, nd.

[178] Porter, 2015b: 79.
[179] Archer, 2003; Bhaskar, 2008; Sayer, 2011.

Chapter 5: Four planes of social being: more connections

[1] Sentamu, 2019; see also Amnesty International, 2018.
[2] Sentamu, 2019.
[3] Gross National Product, the nation's annual income and expenditure.
[4] Greenfield, 2019. The UK pays over £10 billion a year in fossil fuel subsidies, the highest in the EU.
[5] Bhaskar, 2008: 160.
[6] Martin, 2019, and see Chapter 3.
[7] Hills, 2015; Seabrook, 2015; Cooper and Whyte, 2017; CPAG, 2017; Bambra, 2019; Marmot et al, 2020; Marmot, 2015, 2016; and many other references.
[8] https://england.shelter.org.uk/__data/assets/pdf_file/0006/1362885/Findings-The-Impact-of-Housing-Problems-on-Mental-Health.pdf.
[9] Faure Walker, 2019.
[10] Archer, 2003; and see Chapter 3.
[11] Green Hofer, 2020.
[12] Miller and Bauer, 2014; Chang et al, 2011.
[13] Health and Social Care Information Centre, 2013.
[14] RCPsych, 2014.
[15] Green Hofer, 2020.
[16] Green et al, 2016; Green et al, 2018.
[17] Weizenegger, 2020.
[18] Dworkin, 2018.
[19] Taylor and Harvey, 2009.
[20] Tseris, 2013; Wasco, 2003.
[21] Peters, 2019.
[22] Pilgrim, 2002; Melchert, 2015; Benning, 2015; Courtois and Brown, 2019.
[23] Past president of the American Psychiatric Association Steven Sharfstein, 2005: para 5.
[24] Bhaskar et al, 2018.
[25] Collier, 1989; Bhaskar and Danermark, 2006.
[26] Brown, 2018.
[27] Bronfenbrenner, 1979.
[28] Collier, 2005; Danermark et al, 2019.
[29] Sayer, 1992: 119.
[30] Mills, 1956.
[31] Moor and Farchi, 2011.
[32] Owens et al, 2001.
[33] Janoff-Bulman, 1979.
[34] Lerner, 1980.
[35] Suarez and Gadalla, 2010.
[36] Worell and Remer, 2002.
[37] Joyce and Xu, 2019.
[38] Case and Deaton, 2020.
[39] Caused by doctors.
[40] NHS Confederation, 2019.

[41] https://www.theguardian.com/world/2020/may/11/soaring-drug-prices-could-bar-access-to-future-coronavirus-treatments.
[42] Riggs and Greene, 2015; Sainato, 2019.
[43] Paul Johnson, Director of Institute for Fiscal Studies, sponsor of Deaton Report in Joyce and Xu, 2019.
[44] Glasziou and Chalmers, 2009; Macleod et al, 2014; and see Chapter 1.
[45] WOF, 2020.
[46] Interdisciplinarity is far more fully discussed by Bhaskar, 1998 [1979], and Bhaskar et al, 2018.
[47] Durkheim, 1995 [1912].
[48] Bhaskar, 1998 [1979].
[49] Bhaskar et al, 2018: 42–3, adapted from Skinningsrud, 2007.
[50] Bhaskar, 2008; Porpora, 2015.
[51] Adapted from Bhaskar et al, 2018: 14.
[52] Bhaskar and Danermark, 2006: 279.
[53] Midgley, 1996.
[54] Adapted from Bhaskar et al, 2018: 41.
[55] Danermark, 2019.
[56] Alderson et al, 2005; Alderson, 2006.
[57] Fortunately this is the policy in many more ICUs today.
[58] NIDCAP, 2020.
[59] Cochrane Collaboration, www.cochrane.org.
[60] Parker, 2010: 205.
[61] Parker, 2010: 206, citing Fisher and Tronto, 1991: 40.
[62] Porpora, 2015; also see Chapters 4 and 5.
[63] For example, https://bmjopen.bmj.com/content/8/10/e020886; Petterson et al, 2020.
[64] Perera, 2018.
[65] Bhaskar et al, 2018.

Chapter 6: Researching transformative change over time

[1] A composite summary of common problems.
[2] CPAG, 2020.
[3] Catton et al, 2019.
[4] For TMSA, see Chapter 3; Bhaskar, 2008: 53–5; for morphogenesis, see Archer, 1982.
[5] Bhaskar, 2008: 54–5, 392.
[6] Bhaskar, 2008: 299.
[7] Bhaskar, 2010 [1994].
[8] Bhaskar, 2008: 354; Norrie, 2010: 164.
[9] Bhaskar, 2008: 240.
[10] Bhaskar, 2008: 31.
[11] Bhaskar, 2008: 47.
[12] Bhaskar, 2008: 239.
[13] Bhaskar, 2008: 5.
[14] Sartre, 1984.
[15] Shakespeare, *King Lear*, I, i. Lear says this to his third and truthful daughter who refuses to flatter him when he tries to force her to say how much she loves him. She replies, 'nothing', although she really loves and stands by him and unlike her

lying elder sisters she shows the power of self-denying love. In a way, the play grows out of her one word.

[16] Bhaskar, 2008: 48.
[17] Bhaskar, 2008: 396; Norrie, 2010: 23.
[18] Bhaskar, 2010: 8, 2016: 115.
[19] Plato, 1979: 402a.
[20] Norrie, 2010: 207.
[21] Parfit, 1987.
[22] Bhaskar, 2010 [1994]: 119.
[23] Rose and Rose, 2014.
[24] Carey, 2012.
[25] Bhaskar, 2008, 2010 [1994].
[26] Bhaskar, 2016: 115.
[27] Harvey, 2005; Blakeley, 2019: 139–40.
[28] Bhaskar, 2010 [1994]: 11.
[29] Whitehead, 2010: 117.
[30] Derrida, 2016 [1967].
[31] Bhaskar, 2010 [1994]: 14–17.
[32] Bhaskar, 2010 [1994]: 8.
[33] Marx and Engels, 2009 [1845]; Molyneux, 2012: 32–9.
[34] Marx, 1990 [1867]: 102–3.
[35] Marx and Engels, 2009 [1845], summarised by Molyneux, 2012: 32f.
[36] Darwin's evolution of species.
[37] Marx, 1999 [1859]: 389.
[38] Molyneux, 2012: 190–5, criticises Western academics who brought Marxism into disrepute by confusing it with Stalinism, by pursuing ideas and ignoring material realities in the 'Communist' regimes and by misinterpreting Gramsci. They thereby perhaps unintentionally reinforced idealist opposition to Marxism and social justice and led the way into poststructuralism and postmodernism.
[39] Bhaskar, 2016.
[40] Molyneux, 2012: 34.
[41] Bhaskar, 2008: 177.
[42] Including many researchers' dismissal of critical realism.
[43] Bhaskar, 2008 [1975]: 11.
[44] Leigh Price's idea.
[45] Malinowski, 1922; Mead, 1928.
[46] Bhaskar, 2016: 121.
[47] Coleridge, 1834: 175; Keats, 1899, 277; a letter he wrote in 1817.
[48] From Kant's concept of 'conditions of possibility' and 'of possible experience', that things and knowledge rest on prior conditions that make them possible, so that, to understand them, we must first understand these conditions.
[49] Bhaskar, 2008: 205.
[50] Hartwig, 2007: 30-6; Molyneux, 2012: 32–9.
[51] Bhaskar, 2008: 5–8.
[52] Bhaskar, 2008: 282.
[53] Bhaskar, 2008: 309.
[54] Bhaskar, 2008: 125, emphasis in original.
[55] Bhaskar, 2008; Norrie, 2010: 16–18.
[56] Bhaskar, 2008: 125.
[57] Bhaskar, 2008: 208.

[58] Cattermole, 2019.
[59] Bhaskar, 2008: 175.
[60] Bhaskar, 2008: 258.
[61] Bhaskar, 2016: 137.
[62] Bhaskar, 2008: 281.
[63] Bhaskar, 1998 [1979]: 259–62; Archer, 2003; Sayer, 2011.
[64] Arendt, 1986; Bauman, 2005.
[65] Loach and Obiols, 2016.
[66] Willow, 2019.
[67] http://www.restorativejustice4schools.co.uk/wp/?page_id=45
[68] Weinberg, 2020.
[69] Bhaskar, 2008: 201–4.
[70] Bhaskar, 2008: 210.
[71] Bhaskar, 2008: 284–5.
[72] Bhaskar, 2008: 384.
[73] Bhaskar, 2008: 384–5, emphasis in original.
[74] Bhaskar, 2002b: 5–6.
[75] Bhaskar, 2002b: 26.
[76] Mendizabal-Espinosa, 2017.
[77] Marx, 1990 [1867]: 165.
[78] Freud, (1973 [1927]): 147–57.
[79] Case, 2019.
[80] Bhaskar, 2008: 208–9; Molyneux, 2012: 46.
[81] Porter, 2015b: 74.
[82] Mendizabal-Espinosa, 2017, and see Example 2.1 in Chapter 2.
[83] Klaus and Kennell, 1976.
[84] Warner and Spitters, 2017.
[85] RCP, 2003, 2010; Department of Health, 2006; House of Lords Science and Technology Committee, 2007.

Chapter 7: The point is to change it

[1] McKie, 2019.
[2] Garrett, 2019.
[3] https://www.nytimes.com/2019/12/07/health/sickle-cell-adakveo-oxbryta.html
[4] See also Molyneux, 2012.
[5] Pollock, 2004; Davis and Tallis, 2013; Manson, 2013; Davis et al, 2015; El-Gingihy, 2015.
[6] https://lowdownnhs.info/comment/why-bypass-nhs-labs-for-mass-testing-concerns-over-new-super-labs/; https://www.independent.co.uk/news/health/nhs-test-and-trace-mckinsey-management-consultancy-review-a9621351.html; https://yorkshirebylines.co.uk/the-truth-about-the-billion-pound-ppe-procurement-fiasco/; https://www.thecanary.co/uk/analysis/2020/07/11/the-5-5bn-ppe-scandal-that-goes-to-the-core-of-government-incompetence-and-thats-just-for-starters/
[7] Such as Open Democracy, lowdownnhs.info, Keep Our NHS Public, The Canary, Red Revolution.
[8] https://www.theguardian.com/education/2019/sep/03/gove-cummings-dark-arts-education-trash-country
[9] Young and Muller, 2016.

[10] McCoy, 2020.
[11] Burawoy, 2005.
[12] Mackenbach, 2009.
[13] Urry, 2011.
[14] A central aim of critical realism, see Introduction.
[15] Engdahl, 2020.
[16] UN, 1948; UN 1966, 1989.
[17] De Tocqueville, 2000 [1840].
[18] IPCC, 2018.
[19] Shove and Spurling, 2013.
[20] Guterres, 2020.
[21] For example, Independent Commission on a Global Health Risk, 2016.
[22] Centre for Strategic and International Studies, 2019.
[23] Gro Harlem Brundtland, co-chair of the Global Preparedness Monitoring Board, quoted in Garrett, 2019: https://foreignpolicy.com/2019/09/20/the-world-knows-an-apocalyptic-pandemic-is-coming/.
[24] Buranyi, 2020.
[25] Wylie, 2019.
[26] Common Wealth, 2020.
[27] UNCTAD, 2019.
[28] Oxfam, 2020a.
[29] Lynas, 2020.
[30] WHO, 2011.
[31] Davis, 2020.
[32] Lang, 2020.
[33] Blakeley, 2019.
[34] Clark et al, 2020.
[35] Porpora, 2015: 188–208.
[36] Even funds from commercial companies, private trusts and NGOs were originally paid or donated by the general public or are profits from their work.
[37] See Chapter 1.
[38] Abrams, 1968; Mills, 1959.
[39] Adam, 2009: 7.
[40] Urry, 2011.
[41] Wright, 2010.
[42] Unger, 2007.
[43] Levitas, 2013.
[44] Levitas, 2010: 545.
[45] Levitas, 2010.
[46] Harvey, 2012.
[47] D'Souza, 2013: 521. Some of these ideas are drawn from the books D'Souza reviews.
[48] D'Souza, 2013: 520.
[49] D'Souza, 2013: 522, emphasis in original.
[50] From Aristotle's practical wisdom and virtues.
[51] Bhaskar, 2008: 382–3 quoting Marx and Engels, 1998 [1848].
[52] Bhaskar, 2008: 395
[53] Bhaskar, 2002a: 15–16.
[54] Bhaskar, 2008: 296.
[55] Sayer, 2011; D'Souza, 2013.

[56] A reminder that the acronym MELD stands for first Moment, second Edge, third Level and fourth Dimension', see Chapter 6.
[57] Bhaskar, 2008: 382.
[58] Davis, 2020.
[59] Moth, in press.
[60] The terminology used to describe such phenomena is highly contested. Other terms in use include metal illness and mental disorder.
[61] Davies and Bhugra, 2004.
[62] Abbott and Wallace, 1990.
[63] Colombo et al, 2003.
[64] Archer, 1995.
[65] Tew, 2011.
[66] Moth, 2018.
[67] Bhaskar and Danermark, 2006.
[68] Archer, 1995.
[69] Rhodes, 1991.
[70] Bambra et al, 2007: 572.
[71] Bhaskar, 2016.

References

Aadal, L., Angel, S., Dreyer, P., Langhorn, L. and Pedersen, B. B. (2013) Nursing roles and functions in the inpatient of stroke patients: A literature review. *Journal of Neuroscience Nursing*, 45(3): 158–70.

Abbott, P. and Wallace, C. (1990) Social work and nursing: a history. In Abbott, P. and Wallace, C. (eds) *The Sociology of the Caring Professions*. London: Routledge, 10–28.

Abrams, P. (1968) *The Origins of British Sociology: 1834–1914*. Chicago, IL: Chicago University Press.

Adam, B. (2009) Cultural future matters: an exploration in the spirit of Max Weber's methodological writings, *Time & Society*, 18(1): 7–25.

Adhanom Ghebreyesus, T. (2018) *Opening Address at the First WHO Global Conference on Air Pollution and Health*. Geneva: WHO.

Agona, B. (2019) Turning the tide, *The Friend, Quaker Weekly*, 27 September, 26–7.

Aicken, A., Arai, L. and Roberts, H. (2008) *Schemes to Promote Healthy Weight among Obese and Overweight Children in England*. London: EPPI-Centre, University of London.

Alderson, P. (1990) *Choosing for Children: Parents' Consent to Surgery*. Oxford: Oxford University Press.

Alderson, P. (1993) *Children's Consent to Surgery*. Buckingham: Open University Press.

Alderson, P. (1999) Did children change or the guidelines? *Bulletin of Medical Ethics*, 150: 38–44.

Alderson, P. (2006) Parents' consent to neonatal decisions about feeding and discharge, *Journal of Neonatal Nursing*, 12(1): 6–13.

Alderson, P. (2012) Children's consent and 'assent' to health care research. In Freeman, M. (ed) *Law and Childhood Studies*, Oxford University Press, 174–89.

Alderson, P. (2013) *Childhoods Real and Imagined*, vol. 1: *An Introduction to Critical Realism and Childhood Studies*. London: Routledge.

Alderson, P. (2015) Reforms to healthcare systems and policies: influences from children's rights and childhood studies. In Smith, A. (ed.) *Enhancing the Rights and Well-Being of Children: Connecting Research, Policy and Practice*. Basingstoke: Palgrave Macmillan, 17–32.

Alderson, P. (2016) *The Politics of Childhoods Real and Imagined: Practical Application of Critical Realism and Childhood Studies*, vol. 2. London: Routledge.

Alderson, P. and Yoshida, T. (2016) Meanings of children's agency: when and where does agency begin and end? In Esser, F., Baader, M., Betz, T. and Hungerland, B. (eds) *Children as Actors – Childhood and Agency*. London: Routledge, 75–88.

Alderson, P. and Morrow, V. (2020) *The Ethics of Research with Children and Young People: A Practical Handbook*. London: SAGE.

Alderson, P., Killen, M. and Hawthorne, J. (2005) The participation rights of premature babies, *International Journal of Children's Rights*, 13: 31–50.

Alderson, P., Sutcliffe, K. and Curtis, K. (2006a) Children as partners with adults in their medical care, *Archives of Diseases in Childhood*, 91: 300–3.

Alderson, P., Sutcliffe, K. and Curtis, K. (2006b) Children's competence to consent to medical treatment. In *Hastings Centre Report*, 36(6): 25–34.

Alderson, P., Sutcliffe, K. and Mendizabal, R. (2020) A critical realist analysis of consent to surgery for children, human nature and dialectic: the pulse of freedom, *Journal of Critical Realism*, 19(2): 159–71.

Als, H. (1999) Reading the premature infant. In Goldson, E. (ed.) *Developmental Interventions in the Neonatal Intensive Care Nursery*. New York: Oxford University Press, 18–85.

Amnesty International (2018) The Niger Delta is one of the most polluted places on earth, https://www.amnesty.org/en/latest/news/2018/03/Niger-Delta-Oil-Spills-Decoders/

APPG, All-Party Parliamentary Group for Longevity (2019) *The Health of the Nation: A Strategy for Healthier Longer Lives*. London: APPG.

Archer, M. (1982) Morphogenesis versus structuration: on combining structure and agency, *British Journal of Sociology*, 33: 455–83.

Archer, M. (1988) *Culture and Agency: The Place of Culture in Social Theory*. Cambridge: Cambridge University Press.

Archer, M. (1995) *Realist Social Theory: The Morphogenetic Approach*. Cambridge: Cambridge University Press.

Archer, M. (1998) Realism and morphogenesis. In Archer, M., Bhaskar, R., Collier, A., Lawson, T. and Norrie, A. (eds) *Critical Realism: Essential Readings*. London: Routledge, 356–81.

Archer, M. (2000) *Being Human*. Cambridge: Cambridge University Press.

Archer, M. (2003) *Structure, Agency and the Internal Conversation*. Cambridge: Cambridge University Press.

Archer, M. (ed.) (2013) *Social Morphogenesis*. Dordrecht: Springer.

Arendt, H. (1986) *The Origins of Totalitarianism*. London: André Deutsch.

Baker Miller, J. (1976) *Towards a New Psychology of Women*. London: Beacon.
Ball, S. and Head, B. (2020) *Behavioural Insights Teams in Practice: Nudge Missions and Methods on Trial*. Bristol: Policy Press.
Bambra, C. (2016) *Health Divides: Where You Live Can Kill You*. Bristol: Policy Press.
Bambra, C. (2019) *Health in Hard Times: Austerity and Health Inequalities*. Bristol: Policy Press.
Bambra, C., Fox, D. and Scott-Samuel, A. (2007) A politics of health glossary, *Journal of Epidemiology & Community Health*, 61(7): 571–4.
Barber, B. (1962) Resistance by scientists to scientific discovery. In Barber, B. and Hirsch, W. (eds) *The Sociology of Science*. New York: Free Press.
Barnett, A., Campbell, M., Shield, C., Farrington, A., Hall, L., Page, K., Gardner, A., Mitchell, B. and Graves, N. (2016) The high costs of getting ethical and site-specific approvals for multi-centre research, *Research Integrity and Peer Review*, 1(16).
Bartels, S. (2015) Can behavioral health organizations change health behaviors? The STRIDE study and lifestyle interventions for obesity in serious mental illness, *American Journal of Psychology*, 172(1): 9–11.
Bartley, M. (2017) *Health Inequality: An Introduction to Theories, Concepts and Methods*. Cambridge: Polity.
Bashford, A. and Levine, P. (2012) *The Oxford Handbook of the History of Eugenics*. Oxford: Oxford University Press.
Bauman, Z. (2005) *Modernity and the Holocaust*. Cambridge: Polity.
Beauchamp, T. and Childress, J. (2013 [1979]) *Principles of Biomedical Ethics* (7th edn). New York: Oxford University Press.
Beazley, H., Bessell, S., Ennew, E. and Waterson, R. (2009) The right to be properly researched: research with children in a real messy world, *Children's Geographies*, 7(4): 365–78.
Becker, D. (2013) *One Nation under Stress: The Trouble with Stress as an Idea*. Oxford: Oxford University Press.
Belluz, J. (2019) The global crackdown on parents who refuse vaccines for their kids is on, https://www.vox.com/science-and-health/2017/8/3/16069204/vaccine-fines-measles-outbreaks-europe-australia
Benedict, R. (1989) *Patterns of Culture*. Boston, MA: Houghton Mifflin.
Benning T. (2015) Limitations of the biopsychosocial model in psychiatry, *Advances in Medical Education and Practice*, 6:347–52.
Bentham, J. (1988) *The Principles of Morals and Legislation*. Amherst, NY: Prometheus Books.

Bentham, J., Mill, J. and Ryan, A. (1987) *Utilitarianism and Other Essays*. Harmondsworth: Penguin.
Benton, T. (1977) *Philosophical Foundation of the Three Sociologies*. London: Routledge and Kegan Paul.
Bhaskar, R. (1986) *Scientific Realism and Human Emancipation*. London: Routledge.
Bhaskar, R. (1998 [1979]) *The Possibility of Naturalism: A Philosophical Critique of the Contemporary Human Sciences*. London: Routledge.
Bhaskar, R. (2002a) *From Science to Emancipation: Alienation and Enlightenment*. London: Routledge.
Bhaskar, R. (2002b) *Reflection on Meta-Reality: Transcendence, Emancipation and Everyday Life*. London: Routledge.
Bhaskar, R. (2008 [1975]) *A Realist Theory of Science*. London: Routledge.
Bhaskar, R. (2008) *Dialectic: The Pulse of Freedom*. London: Routledge.
Bhaskar, R. (2010 [1994]) *Plato Etc: The Problems of Philosophy and Their Resolution*. London: Routledge.
Bhaskar, R. (2016) *Enlightened Common Sense: The Philosophy of Critical Realism*, edited with a preface by Hartwig, M. London: Routledge.
Bhaskar, R. (2017) *The Order of Natural Necessity. A Kind of Introduction to Critical Realism*, edited by Hawke, G. Amazon.
Bhaskar, R. and Danermark, B. (2006) Metatheory, interdisciplinarity and disability research: a critical realist perspective, *Scandinavian Journal of Disability Research*, 8(4): 278–97.
Bhaskar, R., Danermark, B. and Price, L. (eds) (2018) *Interdisciplinarity and Wellbeing: A Critical Realist General Theory of Interdisciplinarity*. London: Routledge.
Bhumika, Y., Sujeet, G., Yogesh, M. and Devender, P. (2008) Me-too drugs: good or bad? *Pharmaceutical Reviews*, 6(3).
Bissell, P., Thompson, J. and Gibson, B. (2019) Exploring difference or watching the experts at work? *Sociology*, 52: 1200–16.
Blakeley, G. (2019) *Stolen: How to Save the World from Financialisation*. London: Repeater.
Blalock, H. (1969) *Theory Construction from Verbal to Mathematical Formulations*. Upper Saddle River, NY: Prentice Hall.
Blaxter, M. (2000) Class, time and biography. In Williams, S., Gabe, J. and Calnan, M. (eds) *Health, Medicine and Society*. London: Routledge, 27–50.
Bloom, P. (2014) *Just Babies: The Origins of Good and Evil*. New York: Broadway Books.
Boseley, S. (2020a) Coronavirus: UK will have Europe's worst death toll, says study, *Guardian*, 8 April.

Boseley, S. (2020b) Health expert brands UK's coronavirus response 'pathetic', *Guardian*, 12 March.

Boseley, S. (2020c) Neil Ferguson: coronavirus expert who is working on despite symptoms, *Guardian*, 18 March.

Bourdieu, P. (1977) *Outline of a Theory of Practice*. Cambridge: Cambridge University Press.

Bourdieu, P. (1993) *The Field of Cultural Production*. New York: Columbia University Press.

Bourdieu, P. (1998) The essence of neoliberalism, *Le Monde Diplomatique*, December, https://mondediplo.com/1998/12/08bourdieu

Brandenburg, M. (2019) Prescription opioids are associated with population mortality in US deep south middle-age non-Hispanic whites: an ecological time series study, *Frontiers in Public Health*, 06 September, https://doi.org/10.3389/fpubh.2019.00252

Brannan, M., Fleetwood, S., O'Mahoney, J. and Vincent, S. (2017) Meta-analysis: a critical realist critique and alternative, *Human Relations*, 70(1): 11–39.

Broad, K., Curley, J. and Keverne, E. (2006) Mother–infant bonding and the evolution of mammalian social relationships, *Philosophical Transactions*, 361(1476): 2199–214.

Bronfenbrenner, U. (1979) *The Ecology of Human Development: Experiments by Nature and Design*. Cambridge, MA: Harvard University Press.

Brown, L. (2018) *Feminist therapy*. Washington, DC: American Psychological Association.

BSA, British Sociological Association (2003) *Statement of Ethical Practice*. Durham, NC: BSA.

Buranyi, S. (2020) The WHO v coronavirus: why it can't handle the pandemic, *Guardian*, 10 April, https://www.theguardian.com/news/2020/apr/10/world-health-organization-who-v-coronavirus-why-it-cant-handle-pandemic

Burawoy, M. (2005) For public sociology, *American Sociological Review*, 70: 2–28.

Bury, M. (2001) Illness narratives: fact or fiction? *Sociology of Health & Illness*, 23: 263–85.

Butler, J. (2006) *Gender Trouble: Feminism and the Subversion of Identity*. New York: Routledge.

Calnan, M. and Rowe, R. (2008) *Trust Matters in Health Care*. Maidenhead: Open University Press.

Campbell Collaboration (2020) https://www.campbellcollaboration.org.

Carey, N. (2012) *The Epigenetics Revolution: How Modern Biology is Rewriting Our Understanding of Genetics, Disease and Inheritance*. London: Icon.

Case, A. and Deaton, A. (2020) *Deaths of Despair and the Future of Capitalism*. Princeton, NJ: Princeton University Press.

Case, M. (2019) *How to Treat People: A Nurse at Work*. London: Viking.

Cattermole, C. (2019) *Prison: A Survival Guide*. London: Ebury.

Catton, S., Conti, G., Farquharson, C. and Ginja, R. (2019) *The Health Effects of Sure Start*. London: Institute for Fiscal Studies.

Centre for Strategic and International Studies (2019) *Ending the Cycle of Crisis and Complacency in US Global Health Security*. New York: CSIS, UN.

Chalmers, I. (2005) Bill Silverman: a personal appreciation, *Paediatric and Perinatal Epidemiology*, 19(2): 82–5.

Chang, C. K., Hayes, R. D., Perera, G., Broadbent, M., Fernandes, A., Lee, W., Hotopf, M. and Stewart, R. (2011) Life expectancy at birth for people with serious mental illness and other major disorders from a secondary mental health care case register in London. *PLoS ONE*, 6(5): e19590.

Charlie Gard Case (2017) Judgment of the UK Supreme Court in the case of Charlie Gard, 19 June, https://www.supremecourt.uk/cases/docs/charlie-gard-190617.pdf

Charmaz, K. and Bryant, A. (2011) Grounded theory and credibility. In Silverman, D. (ed.) *Qualitative Research: Issues of Theory, Method and Practice*. London: SAGE, 291–309.

Charmaz, K. and Bryant, A. (2019) *The SAGE Handbook of Current Developments in Grounded Theory*. London: SAGE.

Chouliaraki, L. and Fairclough, N. (1999) *Discourse in Late Modernity: Rethinking Critical Discourse Analysis*. Edinburgh: Edinburgh University Press.

Clark, H., Coll-Seck, A., Banerjee, A., Peterson, S., Dalglish, S., et al (2020) A future for the world's children? A WHO–UNICEF–*Lancet* Commission, *The Lancet Commissions*, 395(10224): 605–58.

Clark, M. and Wall, J. (2003) Rehabilitation nursing: The role of the nurse and the development of the specialist role. *Reviews in Clinical Gerontology*, 13(2): 145–52, http://search.ebscohost.com/login.aspx?direct=true&db=rzh&AN=106758958&site=ehost-live.

Clay-Williams, R., Taylor, N. and Braithwaite, J. (2018) Potential solutions to improve the governance of multicentre health services research, *Medical Journal of Australia*, 208(4), 152–4.

Clegg, S. (2005) Evidence-based practice in educational research: a critical realist critique of systematic review, *British Journal of Sociology of Education*, 26(3): 415–28.

Cochrane Collaboration (2020) https://campbell.org.

Coleridge, S. (1834) *Biographia Literaria: Or, Biographical Sketches of My Literary Life and Opinions*. New York: Leavitt, Lord & Co.

Collier, A. (1989) *Scientific Realism and Socialist Thought*. Brighton: Harvester Wheatsheaf.

Collier, A. (1994) *Critical Realism: An Introduction to Bhaskar's Philosophy*. London: Verso.

Collier, A. (2005) Critical realism. In Steinmetz, G. (ed.) *The Politics of Method in the Human Sciences: Positivism and Its Epistemological Others*. London: Duke University Press, 327–45.

Colombo, A., Bendelow, G., Fulford, B. and Williams, S. (2003) Evaluating the influence of implicit models of mental disorder on processes of shared decision making within community-based multi-disciplinary teams, *Social Science & Medicine*, 56(7): 1557–70.

Common Wealth (2020) Blueprint for a new green deal, https://www.common-wealth.co.uk/reports/blueprint-for-a-green-new-deal/

Conn, D. and Lewis, P. (2020) Documents contradict UK government stance on Covid-19 'herd immunity', *Guardian*, 12 April.

Cooper, V. and Whyte, D. (eds) (2017) *The Violence of Austerity*. London: Pluto.

Cornwell, J. (1984) *Hard-Earned Lives*. London: Tavistock.

Corry, M., Porter, S. and McKenna, H. (2019) The redundancy of positivism as a paradigm for nursing research, *Nursing Philosophy*, 20(1): e12230.

Courtois, C. and Brown, L. (2019) Guideline orthodoxy and resulting limitations of the American Psychological Association's Clinical Practice Guideline for the Treatment of PTSD in adults, *Psychotherapy*, 56(3): 329–39.

CPAG, Child Poverty Action Group (2017) *Living Hand to Mouth*. London: CPAG.

CPAG, Child Poverty Action Group (2020) *Child Poverty Facts and Figures*, www.cpag.org.uk/content/child-poverty-facts-and-figures.

CYPMHC, Children and Young People's Mental Health Coalition (nd) *Policy Briefing1: Health Visitors*. London: CYPMHC.

D'Souza, R. (2013) Justice and governance in dystopia, *International Journal of Critical Realism*, 12: 518–37.

Dalkin, S., Greenhalgh, J., Jones, D., Cunningham, B. and Lhussier, M. (2015) What's in a mechanism? Development of a key concept in realist evaluation, *Implementation Science*, 10: 49.

Danermark, B. (2019) Applied interdisciplinary research: a critical realist perspective, *Journal of Critical Realism*, 18(4): 368–82.
Danermark, B., Ekstrom, M. and Karlsson, J. (2019) *Explaining Society: Critical Realism in the Social Sciences*. London: Routledge.
Dasgupta, N., Beletsky, L. and Ciccarone, D. (2018) Opioid crisis: no easy fix to its social and economic determinants, *American Journal of Public Health*, 108(2): 182–6.
Dattani, S. (2020) Why the government changed tack on Covid-19, *Unherd*, 17 March, https://unherd.com/2020/03/the-scientific-case-against-herd-immunity/
Davenport, A. C. (2020) Exploring Nurses' Documentation of their Contribution to Traumatic Brain Injury Rehabilitation in an Aotearoa-New Zealand Rehabilitation Unit. Unpublished PhD thesis. Auckland, New Zealand: Auckland University of Technology.
Davies, D. and Bhugra, D. (2004) *Models of Psychopathology*. Maidenhead: Open University Press.
Davies, W. (2016) *The Happiness Industry: How the Government and Big Business Sold Us Well-Being*. London: Verso.
Davis, C. and Abraham, J. (2013) *Unhealthy Pharmaceutical Regulation: Innovation, Politics and Promissory Science*. Basingstoke: Palgrave Macmillan.
Davis, J. and Tallis, R. (2013) *NHS SOS: How the NHS was Betrayed and How We Can Save it*. London: Oneworld.
Davis, J., Lister, J. and Wrigley, D. (2015) *NHS for Sale: Myths, Lies and Deception*. London: Merlin.
Davis, M. (2020) *COVID-19: The Monster Is at the Door*, Haymarket Books, 12 March.
De Saussure, F. (1983 [1916]) *Course in General Linguistics*. London: Duckworth.
De Tocqueville, A. (2000 [1840]) *Democracy in America*, Vol. 2 (trans and eds H. Mansfield and D. Winthrop). Chicago, IL: University of Chicago Press.
De Vries, J. and Henley, L. (2014) Staying silent when we should speak up: informed consent and the interface between ethics as regulation and ethics in practice. In Posel, D. and Ross, F. C. (eds) *Ethical Quandaries in Social Research*. Cape Town: HSRC Press, 75–92.
De Waal, F. (2013) *The Bonobo and the Atheist: In Search of Humanism among the Primates*. New York: W. W. Norton.
Dean, M. (2013 [1991]) *The Constitution of Poverty*. London: Routledge.
Deleuze, G. and Guattari, F. (1994) *What is Philosophy?* London: Verso.

Denzin, N. and Giardina, M. (eds) (2007) *Ethical Futures in Qualitative Research: Decolonizing the Politics of Knowledge*. Walnut Creek, CA: Left Coast Press.

Department of Health. (2006) A Review of Services for Allergy: The Epidemiology, Demand for and Provision of Treatment and Effective Clinical Interventions. London: Department of Health.

Dermendzhiyska, E. (2020) Cradled by therapy, *AEON*, https://aeon.co/essays/how-attachment-theory-works-in-the-therapeutic-relationship

Derrida, J. (2016 [1967]) *Of Grammatology*. Baltimore, ML: Johns Hopkins University Press.

DfE, Department for Education (2019) *A Guide to Looked After Children Statistics in England*. London: DfE.

Dingwall, R. (2008) The ethical case against ethical regulation in humanities and social science research, *Twenty-First Century Society*, 3: 1–12.

Dingwall, R. (2018) How did we ever get into this mess? Ethics in social research, *Studies in Qualitative Methodology*, 12: 3–26.

Dixon-Woods, M. (2011) Systematic reviews and qualitative methods. In Silverman, D. (ed.) *Qualitative Research: Issues of Theory, Method and Practice*. London: SAGE, 331–46.

Dorling, D. (2013) *Unequal Health: The Scandal of our Times*. Bristol: Policy Press.

Dorling, D. (2015) Comment. Income inequality and health: a causal review, *Social Science & Medicine*, 128: 316–26.

Dorling, D. (2020) Foreword. In O'Hara, M. (ed.) *The Shame Game: Overturning the Toxic Poverty Narrative*. Bristol: Policy Press, xiii–xvi.

Dorling, D. and Thomas, B. (2009) Geographical inequalities in health over the last century. In Graham, H. (ed.) *Understanding Health Inequalities*. Buckingham: Open University Press, 66–83.

Doshi, P. (2020) WHO's malaria vaccine study represents a 'serious breach of international ethical standards', *British Medical Journal*, 368: m734, https://doi.org/10.1136/bmj.m734.

Drew, P., Chatwin, J. and Collins, S. (2008) Conversation analysis: a method for research into interactions between patients and health-care professionals, *Health Expectations*, 4: 58–70.

Dummer, T. (2008) Health geography: supporting public health policy and planning, *Canadian Medial Association Journal*, 178(9): 1177–80.

Durkheim, E. (1995 [1912]) *The Elementary Forms of Religious Life* (trans. K. Fields). New York: Free Press.

Dworkin, E. (2018) Risk for mental disorders associated with sexual assault: a meta-analysis, *Trauma, Violence and Abuse*, 21(5): 1011–28, https://doi.org/10.1177/1524838018813198

Edwards, P., O'Mahony, J. and Vincent, S. (2014a) Concluding comments. In Edwards, P., O'Mahony, J. and Vincent, S. (eds) *Studying Organizations Using Critical Realism: A Practical Guide*. Oxford: Oxford University Press, 318–26.

Edwards, P., O'Mahony, J. and Vincent, S. (eds) (2014b) *Studying Organizations Using Critical Realism: A Practical Guide*. Oxford: Oxford University Press.

Edwards, R. and Mauthner, M. (2012) Ethics and feminist research: theory and practice. In Miller, T., Birch, M., Mauthner, M. and Bishop, J. (eds) *Ethics in Qualitative Research*. London: SAGE, 14–28.

El-Gingihy, Y. (2015) *How To Dismantle the NHS in 10 Easy Steps*. Aylesford: Zero Books.

Eliot, G. (1994 [1874]) *Middlemarch*. Harmondsworth: Penguin.

Ellis-Peterson, H. (2019) Five million pollution masks to be handed to Delhi residents, *Guardian*, 2 November.

Engdahl, F. (2020) Coronavirus, vaccines and the Gates Foundation, *Global Research*, 20 March, https://www.globalresearch.ca/coronavirus-gates-foundation/5706842?print=1.

ESRC, Economic and Social Research Council (2005) *Research Ethics Framework*. Swindon: ESRC.

Farsides, T. and Sparks, P. (2016) Buried in bullshit, *The Psychologist*, 29: 368–71.

Faure Walker, R. (2019) The UK's PREVENT counter-terrorism strategy appears to promote rather than prevent violence, *Journal of Critical Realism*, 18(5): 487–512.

Felbab-Brown, V. (2019) *The U.S. Opioid Epidemic and Lessons for the World*. Las Vegas, NV: Brookings Institution, https://digitalscholarship.unlv.edu/brookings_lectures_events/145/

Fisher, B. and Tronto, J. (1991) Toward a feminist theory of care. In Abel, E. and Nelson, M. (eds) *Circles of Care*. Albany, NY: SUNY Press, 36–54.

Fisher, M. (2009) *Capitalist Realism: Is There No Alternative?* Aylesford: Zero Books.

Fonagy, P. (2001) *Attachment Theory and Psychoanalysis*. New York: Other Press.

Ford, M. (2020) *The Government Is Treading a Dangerous Path in Its Response to Covid-19*. London: Centre for Crime and Justice Studies.

Formosa, M. and Higgs, P. (2013) *Social Class in Later Life: Power, Identity and Life Style*. Bristol: Policy Press.

Foucault, M. (1963) *Birth of the Clinic*. New York: Pantheon.
Foucault, M. (1977) *Discipline and Punish*. New York: Random House.
Fox, N. (2011) The ill-health assemblage: beyond the body-with-organs, *Health Sociology Review*, 20(4): 359–71.
Fox, R. (2008) The bioethics I would like to see, *Clinical Ethics*, 3: 25–6.
Frank, A. (1995) *The Wounded Storyteller: Body, Illness and Ethics*. Chicago, IL: University of Chicago Press.
Freud, S. (1973 [1927]). Fetishism. In J. Strachey (ed.) *The Standard Edition of the Complete Psychological Works of Sigmund Freud*, vol. 21. London: Hogarth Press, 152–9.
Garfinkel, H. (1984) Studies in *Ethnomethodology*. Cambridge: Polity.
Garrett, L. (2019) The world knows an apocalyptic pandemic is coming, but nobody is interested in doing anything about it, *Foreign Policy*, 20 September, https://foreignpolicy.com/2019/09/20/the-world-knows-an-apocalyptic-pandemic-is-coming/
Garthwaite, K. (2017) *Hunger Pains*. Bristol: Policy Press.
Garthwaite, K. and Bambra, C. (2017) 'How the other half live': lay perspectives on health inequalities in an age of austerity, *Social Science & Medicine*, 187: 268–75.
Gaventa, J. and Cornwall, A. (2008) *Power and Knowledge*. London: SAGE.
Gearty, C. (2011) About the project, http://therightsfuture.com/about/
Geertz, C. (1984) Culture and social change: the Indonesian case, *Man*, 19: 511–32.
Giddens, A. (1979) *Central Problems in Social Theory*. Basingstoke: Macmillan.
Glaser, B. and Strauss, A. (1965) *Awareness of Dying*. Chicago, IL: Aldine.
Glaser, B. and Strauss, A. (1967) *The Discovery of Grounded Theory*. Chicago, IL: Aldine.
Glasziou, P. and Chalmers, I. (2009) Avoidable waste in the production and reporting of research evidence, *Lancet*, 374(9683): 86–9.
Glynos, J., Speed, E. and West, K. (2015) Logics of marginalisation in health and social care reform: integration, choice and provider-blind provision, *Critical Social Policy*, 35(1): 45–68.
Gobo, G. (2011) Ethnography. In Silverman, D. (ed.) *Qualitative Research: Issues of Theory, Method and Practice*. London: SAGE, 15–34.
Goffman, A. (2014) *On the Run: Fugitive Life in an American City*. Chicago, IL: University of Chicago Press.
Goffman, E. (1959) *The Presentation of the Self in Everyday Life*. Edinburgh: University of Edinburgh Press.

Goffman, E. (1961) *Asylums: Essays on the Social Situation of Mental Patients and Other Inmates*. New York: Doubleday.

Goldacre, B. (2012) *Bad Pharma: How Medicine is Broken, And How We Can Fix It*. London: Fourth Estate.

Goldacre, B. (2018) *I Think You'll Find It's a Bit More Complicated than That*. London: Fourth Estate.

Goodfield, J. (1981) *An Imagined World*. New York: Harper & Row.

Gopnik, A. (2010) *The Philosophical Baby: What Children's Minds Tell Us About Truth, Love, and the Meaning of Life*. London: Picador.

Gorski, P. (2013) What is critical realism and why should you care? *Contemporary Sociology*, 42(5): 658–70.

Gough, D., Oliver, S. and Thomas, J. (2018) *Systematic Reviews and Research*. London: SAGE.

Gouldner, A. (1977) *The Coming Crisis in Western Sociology*. London: Routledge.

Green Hofer, S. (2020) Complexity, co-creation and social practices – re-constructing quality improvement: a case study in mental health. PhD thesis. London: London School of Hygiene and Tropical Medicine.

Green, S., Evans, L., Matthews, R., et al (2016) Service user engagement in quality improvement: applying the national involvement standards, *Journal of Mental Health Training and Education Practice*, 11(5): 279–85.

Green, S. et al (2018) Implementing guidelines on physical health in the acute mental health setting: a quality improvement approach, *International Journal of Mental Health*, 12(1), https://doi.org/10.1186/s13033-018-0179-1

Greenfield, P. (2019) World's top three asset managers oversee $300bn fossil fuel investment, *Guardian*, 12 October.

Greenhalgh, J. (2014) Realist synthesis. In Edwards, P., O'Mahony, J. and Vincent, S. (eds) *Studying Organizations Using Critical Realism: A Practical Guide*. Oxford: Oxford University Press, 264–81.

Greenhalgh, T., Wong, G., Jagosh, J., Greenhalgh, J., Manzano, A., Westhorp, G. and Pawson, R. (2015) Protocol—the RAMESES II study: developing guidance and reporting standards for realist evaluation, *BMJ Open*, 5(8): e008567.

Guba, Y. and Lincoln, E. (1989) *Fourth Generation Evaluation*. London: SAGE.

Guba, Y. and Lincoln, E. (1992) *Effective Evaluation*. San Francisco, CA: Jossey-Bass.

Guterres, A. (2020) UN secretary general: recovery from the coronavirus crisis must lead to a better world, *Guardian*, 2 April.

Haben, G. (2019) *The Deafblind Woman Who Conquered Harvard Law*. New York: Grand Central Publishing.

Habermas, J. (1987) *The Theory of Communicative Action*, Vol. 2. Cambridge: Polity.

Hall, D. and Hall, S. (2007) *The 'Family-Nurse Partnership': Developing an Instrument for Identification, Assessment and Recruitment of Clients*. London: Department for Children, Schools and Families.

Hammersley, M. (1995) *The Politics of Social Research*. London: SAGE.

Hammersley, M. and Traianou, A. (2014) An alternative ethics? Justice and care as guiding principles for qualitative research, *Sociological Review Online*, 19: 24.

Hartwig, M. (2007) *Dictionary of Critical Realism*. London: Routledge.

Harvey, D. (2005) *A Brief History of Neoliberalism*. Chicago, IL: University of Chicago Press.

Harvey, D. (2012) Hardtalk interview, BBC World Service, 12 July, https://www.youtube.com/watch?v=zARceZS50ps

Hayes, B., Bonner, A. and Pryor, J. (2010) Factors contributing to nurse job satisfaction in the acute hospital setting: A review of recent literature. *Journal of Nursing Management*, 18(7): 804–14, http://search.ebscohost.com/login.aspx?direct=true&db=rzh&AN=2010828013&site=ehost-live.

Health and Social Care Information Centre (2013) *Mental Health Bulletin: Annual Report from MHMDS Returns—England 2011–2012*. Leeds: HSCIC.

Hedgecoe, A. (2016) Reputational risk, academic freedom and research ethics review, *Sociology*, 3: 486–501.

Hérbert and Rosen, W. (2019) *Doing Right: A Practical Guide to Ethics for Medical Trainees and Physicians*. New York: Oxford University Press.

Hewlett, B. and Hewlett, B. (2008) *Ebola, Culture and Politics: The Anthropology of an Emerging Disease*. Belmont, CA: Thomson Wadsworth.

Hills, J. (2015) *Good Times, Bad Tines: The Welfare Myth of Them and Us*. Bristol: Policy Press.

Hinds, K. and Dickson, K. (in press) Realist synthesis: A critique and an alternative, *International Journal of Critical Realism*.

Holmwood, J. (2010) Research ethics committees (RECs) and the creaking piers of peer review, *Sociological Research Online*, 15(4): 14.

Holmwood, J. (2014) From social rights to the market: neoliberalism and the knowledge economy, *International Journal of Lifelong Education*, 33: 62–76.

Horton, R. (2020) Offline: COVID-19 and the NHS—'a national scandal', *Lancet*, 395(10229): 1022.

House of Lords Science and Technology Committee (2007) Allergy, Sixth Report of Session 2006–2007. London: House of Lords.

Huang, C. et al (2020) Clinical features of patients infected with 2019 novel coronavirus in Wuhan, China, *Lancet*, 395(10223): 497–506, https://doi.org/10.1016/S0140-6736(20)30183-5

Hughes, G. (2017) New models of care: the policy discourse of integrated care, *People, Place & Policy*, 11(2): 72–89.

Hume, D. (1739) *A Treatise of Human Nature*. London: John Noon.

Hume, D. (1748) *An Enquiry Concerning Human Understanding*. Edinburgh.

Independent Commission on a Global Health Risk (2016) *The Neglected Dimension of Global Security: A Framework to Counter Infectious Disease Crises. Framework for the Future.* Washington, DC: National Academy of Medicine.

INVOLVE (2012) *Briefing Notes for Researchers: Involving the Public in NHS, Public Health and Social Care Research*. Eastleigh: INVOLVE.

Ioannidis, J. (2016) Why most clinical research is not useful, *PLoS Medicine*, 13(6): e1002049.

IPCC, Intergovernmental Panel on Climate Change (2018) Global warming of 1.5°, https://report.ipcc.ch/sr15/pdf/sr15_spm_final.pdf

Israel, M. (2018) Ethical imperialism? Exporting research ethics to the Global South. In Iphofen, R. and Tolich, M. (eds) *The SAGE Handbook of Qualitative Research Ethics*. London: SAGE, 90–113.

Janoff-Bulman, R. (1979) Characterological vs behavioural self-blame: inquiries into depression and rape, *Journal of Personality and Social Psychology*, 37(10): 1798–809.

Janzen, S. K. and Mugler, A. N. (2009) Expanding the scope of staff education: Brain injury to polytrauma. *Rehabilitation Nursing*, 34(5): 181, http://search.ebscohost.com/login.aspx?direct=true&db=rzh&AN=2010403260&site=ehost-live.

Jinks, A. M. and Hope, P. (2000) What do nurses do? An observational survey of the activities of nurses on acute surgical and rehabilitation wards. *Journal of Nursing Management*, 8(5): 273–9.

Joyce, R. and Xu, X. (2019) *Are the Inequalities Seen Today a Sign of a Broken System? Launch of the IFS Deaton Review of inequalities*. London: Institute for Fiscal Studies.

Kant, I. (1964) *Metaphysic of Morals*, part 2, trans. Gregor, M. London: Harper Row.

Keats, J. (1899) *The Complete Poetical Works and Letters of John Keats*. Boston, MA: Houghton, Mifflin and Company.

Keller, E. (1985) *Reflections on Gender and Science*. New Haven, CT: Yale University Press.

Kim, J., Alderete, T., Chen, Z., Lurmann, F., Rappaport, E., Habre, R., Berhane, K. and Gilliland, F. (2018) Longitudinal associations of *in utero* and early life near-roadway air pollution with trajectories of childhood body mass index, *Environmental Health*, 17: 64.

Kirkpatrick, T. et al (2018) Evaluation of a complex intervention (Engager) for prisoners with common mental health problems, near to and after release: study protocol for a randomised controlled trial, *BMJ Open*, https://doi: 10.1136/bmjopen-2017-017931, see Engager site: https://www.plymouth.ac.uk/research/primarycare/engager

Klaus, M. and Kennell, J. (1976) *Maternal-Infant Bonding*. St Louis, MO: C. Moseby.

Klein, N. (2007) *The Shock Doctrine: The Rise of Disaster Capitalism*. London: Penguin.

Kleinman, A., Das, V. and Lock, M. (1997) *Social Suffering*. Berkeley, CA: University of California Press.

Knox, H. (2019) Fat shaming vs fat empowerment: the construction of fat bodies in neoliberal discourse, *Cultivate, The Feminist Journal of the Centre for Women's Studies* (no pages).

Koç, A. (2012). Rehabilitation nursing: Applications for rehabilitation nursing. *International Journal of Caring Sciences*, 5(2): 6.

Krieger, N. (1994) Epidemiology and the web of causation: has anyone seen the spider? *Social Science & Medicine*, 39(7): 887–903.

Krieger, N. (2008) Proximal, distal, and the politics of causation: what's level got to do with it? *American Journal of Public Health*, 98(2): 221–30.

Kruk, M., Gage, A., Joseph, N., Danaei, G., Garcia-Saiso, S. and Salomon, J. (2018) Mortality due to low-quality health systems in the universal health coverage era: a systematic analysis of amenable deaths in 137 countries, *Lancet*, 392(10160): 2203–12.

Kuhn, T. (2017 [1962]) *The Structure of Scientific Revolutions*. Chicago, IL: Chicago University Press.

Kurtz, Z., McLeish, J., Arora, A. and Ball, M. (2005) *Maternity Services Provision in Sure Start Local Programmes*. London: Department for Education and Skills.

Lang, T. (2020) *Feeding Britain*. London: Pelican.

Latour, B. (2007) *Reassembling the Social: An Introduction to Actor Network Theory*. Oxford: Oxford University Press.

Law, J. (2009) Actor network theory and material semiotics. In Turner, B. (ed.) *The New Blackwell Companion to Social Theory*. New York: Wiley Blackwell, 141–58.

Lawson, T. (1998) Economic science without experimentation. In Archer, M., Bhaskar, R., Collier, A., Lawson, T. and Norrie, A. (eds) *Critical Realism: Essential Readings*. London: Routledge, 144–69.

Layard, R. (2011) *Happiness: Lessons from a New Science*. London: Penguin.
Leiter, K. (1980) *A Primer of Ethnomethodology*. Oxford: Oxford University Press.
Lerner, M. (1980) *The Belief in a Just World: A Fundamental Delusion*. New York: Plenum.
Levitas, R. (2010) Back to the future: wells, sociology, utopia and method, *Sociological Review*, 58: 530–47.
Levitas, R. (2013) *Utopia as Method: The Imaginary Reconstitution of Society*. Basingstoke: Palgrave Macmillan.
Lincoln, Y. (1995) Emerging criteria for quality in qualitative and interpretive inquiry, *Qualitative Inquiry*, 1(3): 275–89.
Loach, K. (2019) *Sorry We Missed You*. Entertainment One, UK.
Loach, K. and Obiols (2016) *I, Daniel Blake*. Sixteen Films, UK.
Locke, J. (1959) *An Essay Concerning Human Understanding*, Vol. 1. New York: Dover.
Lowe, P., Lee, E. and Mavarish, J. (2015) Biologising parenting: neuroscience discourse, English social and public health policy and understandings of the child, *Sociology of Health and Illness*, 37(2): 198–211.
Lukes, S. (2005) *Power: A Radical View*. Basingstoke: Palgrave Macmillan.
Lukes, S. (2008) *Moral Relativism*. London: Profile.
Lynas, M. (2020) *Our Final Warning: Six Degrees of Climate Emergency*. Glasgow: Harper Collins.
Lynch, M. (1993) *Scientific Practice and Ordinary Action: Ethnomethodology and Social Studies of Science*. Cambridge: Cambridge University Press.
MacIntyre, A. (2007 [1981]) *After Virtue: A Study in Moral Theory*. Indiana, IN: University of Notre Dame Press.
Mackenbach, J. (2009) Politics is nothing but medicine at a larger scale: reflections on public health's biggest idea, *Journal of Epidemiology & Community Health*, 63: 181–4.
Macklin, R. (2003) Dignity is a useless concept, *British Medical Journal*, 327: 1419–20.
Macleod, M., Michie, S., Roberts, I., Dirnagl, U., Chalmers, I., Ioannidis, J., Salman, R., Chan, A.-W. and Glasziou, P. (2014) Biomedical research: increasing value, reducing waste, *Lancet*, 383(9912): 101–4.
Malinowski, B. (1922) *Argonauts of the Western Pacific: An account of native enterprise and adventure in the Archipelagoes of Melanesian New Guinea*. London: Routledge and Kegan Paul.

Manson, J. (ed.) (2013) *Public Service on the Brink*. Exeter: Imprint Academic.

Manyukhina, Y. (2018) *Ethical Consumption: Practices and Identities: A Realist Approach*. London: Routledge.

Marchal, B., van Belle, S., van Olmen, J., Hoerée, T. and Kegels, G. (2012) Is realist evaluation keeping its promise? A review of published empirical studies in the field of health systems research, *Evaluation*, 18(2): 192–212.

Marmot, M. (2015) *Status Syndrome: How Your Place on the Social Gradient Directly Affects Your Health*. London: Bloomsbury.

Marmot, M. (2016) *The Health Gap: The Challenge of an Unequal World*. London: Bloomsbury.

Marmot, M., Allen, J., Boyce, T., Goldblatt, P. and Morrison, J. (2020) *Health Equity in England: The Marmot Review 10 Years On*. London: Institute of Health Equity.

Marteau, T. (2018) Changing minds about changing behaviour, *Lancet*, 391(10116): 116–17.

Martin, K. (2019) A critical realist study of shared decision-making in young people's mental health inpatient units. PhD thesis. London: University College London.

Martin, R. and Barresi, J. (2006) *The Rise and Fall of the Soul and Self: An Intellectual History of Personal Identity*. New York: Columbia University Press.

Marx, K. and Engels, F. (2009 [1845]) *The Roots of the Socialist Philosophy: Theses on Feuerbach*. (trans. A. Lewis). New York: Mondial.

Marx, K. (1999 [1859]) Preface to *A Contribution to the Critique of Political Economy* (trans. T. Delaney). Oakham, UK: Zodiac.

Marx, K. (1990 [1867]) *Capital* (trans. B. Fowkes). London: Penguin.

Marx, K. (2000 [1852]) The eighteenth Brumaire of Louis Bonapart. In McClellan, D. (ed.) *Karl Marx, Selected Writings*. New York: Oxford University Press, 300–25.

Marx, K. and Engels, F. (1998 [1848]) *Communist Manifesto*. London: Penguin.

McCarraher, E. (2019) *The Enchantments of Mammon: How Capitalism Became the Religion of Modernity*. Cambridge, MA: Harvard University Press.

McCoy, D. (2020) Faith in coronavirus modelling is no substitute for sound political judgment, *Guardian*, 10 April.

McDonnell, O. (2013) Social constructionism. In Gabe, J. and Monaghan, L. (eds) *Key Concepts in Medical Sociology*. London: SAGE, 130–4.

McKeown, T. (1976) *The Role of Medicine*. London: Nuffield.

McKie, R. (2019) 'We can beat Ebola but must prepare for what comes next,' says Wellcome Trust head, *Observer*, 22 December.

Mead, M. (1928) *Coming of Age in Samoa*. London: William Morrow.

Melchert, T. (2015) *Biopsychosocial Practice: A Science Based Framework for Behavioural Healthcare*. Washington, D.C.: American Psychological Association.

Mendizabal-Espinosa, R. (2017) A critical realist study of neonatal intensive care in Mexico. PhD thesis. London: University College London.

Mendizabal-Espinosa, R. and Warren, I. (2019) Non-evidence-based beliefs increase inequalities in the provision of infant- and family-centred neonatal care, *Acta Paediatrica*, 109(2): 314–20, https://doi:10.1111/apa.14972

Merson, A. (2020) Professor Hugh Pennington: 'Herd immunity is a crazy idea, not really supported by any sound science', *The Press and Journal*, 23 March, https://www.pressandjournal.co.uk/fp/news/politics/uk-politics/2093482/professor-hugh-pennington-herd-immunity-is-a-crazy-idea-not-really-supported-by-any-sound-science/

Mertens, D., Holmes, H. and Harris, R. (2009) Transformative research and ethics. In Mertens, D. and Ginsberg, P. (eds) *Handbook of Research Ethics*. Thousand Oaks, CA: SAGE, 85–103.

Metz, T. (2013) The Western ethic of care or an Afro-communitarian ethic? Specifying the right relational morality, *Journal of Global Ethics*, 9(1): 77–92.

Midgley, M. (1994) *The Ethical Primate*. London: Routledge.

Midgley, M. (1996) *Utopias, Dolphins and Computer: Problems of Philosophical Plumbing*. London: Routledge.

Midgley, M. (2002) *Beast and Man: The Roots of Human Nature*. London: Routledge.

Miller, C. and Bauer, M. (2014) Excess mortality in bipolar disorders, *Current Psychiatry Reports*, 16(11): 499.

Miller, J. and Glassner, B. (2011) The 'inside' and the 'outside': finding reality in interviews. In Silverman, D. (ed.) *Qualitative Research: Issues of Theory, Method and Practice*. London: SAGE, 131–48.

Mills, C. W. (1956) *The Power Elite*. New York: Oxford University Press.

Mills, C. W. (1959) *The Sociological Imagination*. New York: Oxford University Press.

Mindfulness and Social Change Network (2020) https://mindfulnessandsocialchange.org/

Mire, S. (2020) *Divine Fertility: The Continuity in Transformation of an Ideology of Sacred Kinship in North-East Africa*. London: UCL Institute of Archaeology Publications.

Mirowski, P. (2014) *Never Let a Serious Crisis Go to Waste: How Neoliberalism Survived the Financial Meltdown*. London: Verso.

Mirowski, P. and Plehwe, D. (eds) (2009) *The Road from Mont Pelerin: The Making of the Neoliberal Thought Collective*. Cambridge, MA: Harvard University Press.

Mogre, V., Scherpbier, A., Stevens, F., Aryee, P., Cherry, A. and Dornan, T. (2016) Realist synthesis of educational interventions to improve nutrition care competencies and delivery by doctors and other healthcare professionals, *BMJ Open*, 6: e010084.

Mol, A. (2003) *The Body Multiple: Ontology in Medical Practice*. Durham, NC: Duke University Press.

Molyneux, J. (2012) *The Point Is to Change It!* London: Bookmarks.

Moynihan, R. and Cassels, A. (2005) *Selling Sickness: How the World's Biggest Pharmaceutical Companies Are Turning Us All into Patients*. Vancouver: Greystone Books.

Moor, A. and Farchi, M. (2011) Is rape-related self blame distinct from other post traumatic attributions of blame? A comparison of severity and implications for treatment, *Women and Therapy*, 34(4): 447–60.

Morgan, J. (2007) Mind. In Hartwig, M. (ed.) *Dictionary of Critical Realism*. London: Routledge, 314–15.

Morreira, S. (2012) Anthropological futures? Thoughts on social research and the ethics of engagement, *Anthropology Southern Africa*, 35: 100–4.

Moth, R. (2018) 'The business end': neoliberal policy reforms and biomedical residualism in frontline community mental health practice in England, *Competition & Change*, 24(2), 133–53.

Moth, R. (in press) *Understanding Mental Distress: Knowledge, Practice and Neoliberal Reform in Community Mental Health Services*. Bristol: Policy Press.

MRC, Medical Research Council (1964) Responsibility in investigations on human subjects. In *Annual Report (1962–3)*. London: HMSO, 21–5.

Murphy, M. (2017) *The Economization of Life*. Durham, NC: Duke University Press.

NAO, National Audit Office (2020) *Information Held by the Department for Work & Pensions on Deaths by Suicide of Benefit Claimants*. London: NAO.

National Commission for the Protection of Human Subjects of Biomedical and Behavioral Research (1979) *Belmont Report: Ethical Principles and Guidelines for the Protection of Human Subjects of Research*. Washington, DC: DHSS, Federal Register.

Navarro, V. (2020) The consequences of neoliberalism in the current pandemic, *International Journal of Health Services*, 50(3), 271–5, https://doi.org/10.1177/0020731420925449

Neel, K., Goldman, R., Marte, D., Bello, G. and Nothnagle, M. (2019) Hospital-based maternity care practitioners' perceptions of doulas, *Birth: Issues in Perinatal Care*, 46: 355–61, https://doi.org/10.1111/birt.12420

NHS Confederation (2019) *The NHS and Future Free Trade Agreements*. London: NHS Confederation, 22 October.

NIDCAP, Newborn Individualized Developmental Care and Assessment Program (2020) www.nidcap.org

Norrie, A. (2010) *Dialectic and Difference: Dialectical Critical Realism and the Grounds of Justice*. London: Routledge.

NRLS, National Reporting and Learning System (2019) https://report.nrls.nhs.uk/nrlsreporting/

Nuremberg Code (1947) http://www.cirp.org/library/ethics/nuremberg/.

Nussbaum, M. (1999) Virtue ethics: a misleading category? *Journal of Ethics*, 3(3): 163–201.

Nussbaum, M. (2006) *Frontiers of Justice*. Cambridge, MA: Harvard University Press.

O'Hara, M. (2020) *The Shame Game: Overturning the Toxic Poverty Narrative*. Bristol: Policy Press.

Oakley, A. (1981) Interviewing women: a contradiction in terms? In Roberts, H. (ed.) *Doing Feminist Research*. London: Routledge, 30–61.

Oliver, M. (2009) *Understanding Disability: From Theory to Practice*. Basingstoke: Macmillan.

Oswell, D. (2012) *The Agency of Children: From Family to Global Human Rights*. Cambridge: Cambridge University Press.

Owens, G., Pike, J. and Chard, K. (2001) Treatment effects of cognitive processing therapy on cognitive distortions of female child sexual abuse survivors, *Behaviour Therapy*, 32(3): 413–24.

Oxfam (2020a) *Dignity Not Destitution: An 'Economic Rescue Plan For All ' to Tackle the Coronavirus Crisis and Rebuild a More Equal World*. Oxford: Oxfam.

Oxfam (2020b) World's billionaires have more wealth than 4.6 billion people, https://www.oxfam.org/en/press-releases/worlds-billionaires-have-more-wealth-46-billion-people

Paine, T. (2000 [1791]) *The Rights of Man*. London: Dover Publications.

Pappworth, M. (1967) *Human Guinea Pigs: Experimentation on Man*. London: Routledge.

Parfit, D. (1987) Divided minds and the nature of persons. In Blakemore, C. and Greenfield, S. (eds) *Mindwaves*. Oxford: Blackwell, 19–26.

Parker, J. (2010) Towards a dialectics of knowledge and care in the global system. In Bhaskar, R., Frank, C., Hoyer, K., Næss, P. and Parker, J. (eds) (2010) *Interdisciplinarity and Climate Change*. London: Routledge, 205–26.

Parsons, T. (1951) *The Social System*. Glencoe, IL: Free Press.

Pauli, B. (2019) *Flint Fight Back: Environmental Justice and Democracy in the Flint Water Crisis*. Cambridge, MA: MIT Press.

Pawson, R. (2006) *Evidence-Based Policy: A Realist Perspective*. London: SAGE.

Pawson, R. (2013) *The Science of Evaluation: A Realist Manifesto*. London: SAGE.

Pawson, R. (2016a) Realist evaluation caricatured: a reply to Porter, *Nursing Philosophy*, 17(2): 132–9.

Pawson, R. (2016b) The ersatz realism of critical realism: a reply to Porter, *Evaluation*, 22(1): 49–57.

Pawson, R. and Tilley, N. (1997) *Realistic Evaluation*. London: SAGE.

Pawson, R. and Manzano-Santaella, A. (2012) A realist diagnostic workshop, *Evaluation*, 18(2): 176–91.

Pawson, R., Greenhalgh, T., Harvey, G. and Walshe, K. (2005) Research review: a new method of systematic review designed for complex policy interventions, *Journal of Health Service Policy*, 10(S1): 21–34.

Pearce, F. (2007) *When the Rivers Run Dry: What Happens When Our Water Runs Out?* London: Eden Project.

Pellegrino, E. and Thomasma, D. (1994) *The Virtues in Medical Practice*. Oxford: Oxford University Press.

Penn, R. and Kiddy, M. (2011) MMR: factors for uptake, *Community Practitioner*, 84(11): 42–3.

Perera, F. (2018) Pollution from fossil-fuel combustion is the leading environmental threat to global pediatric health and equity: solutions exist, *International Journal of Environmental Research and Public Health*, 15(1): 16.

Peters, S. M. (2019) Demedicalising the aftermath of sexual assault: toward a radical humanistic approach, *Journal of Humanistic Psychology*, https://doi:10.1177/0022167819831526

Petterson, S., Westfall, J. and Miller, B. (2020) *Projected Deaths of Despair during the Coronavirus Recession*. California: Well Being Trust.

Pettigrew, M. and Davey Smith, G. (2012) The monkey puzzle: a systematic review of studies of stress, social hierarchies, and heart disease in monkeys, *PLoS ONE*, 7(3): e27939, https://doi:10.1371/journal.pone.0027939

Pierrat, V., Coquelin, A., Cuttini, M., Khoshnood, B., Glorieux, I., Claris, O., Durox, M., Kaminski, M., Ancel, P.-Y. and Arnaud, C. (2016) Translating neurodevelopmental care policies into practice, *Pediatric Critical Care Medicine*, 17(10): 957–67.

Pilgrim, D. (2002) The biopsychosocial model in Anglo-American psychiatry: past, present and future? *Journal of Mental Health*, 11(6): 585–94.

Pilnick, A. and Dingwall, R. (2011) On the remarkable persistence of asymmetry in doctor/patient interaction: a critical review, *Social Science & Medicine*, 72(8): 1374–82.

Place, B. (2000) Constructing the bodies of critically ill children: an ethnography of intensive care. In Prout, A. (ed.) *The Body, Childhood and Society*. Basingstoke: Macmillan, 172–94.

Plato (1979) Cratylus. In Cooper, J. (ed.) *Plato: Complete Works*. Indianapolis, IN: Hackett.

Plato (2019) *The Republic*. London: Penguin Classics.

Polanyi, K. (1944) *The Great Transformation*. Boston, MA: Beacon.

Pollock, A. (2004) *NHS PLC: The Privatisation of Our Health Care*. London: Verso.

Popper, K. (1945 [2011]) *The Open Society and its Enemies*. London: Routledge.

Porpora, D. (1998) Four concepts of social structure. In Archer, M., Bhaskar, R., Collier, A., Lawson, A. and Norrie, A. (eds) *Critical Realism Essential Readings*. London: Routledge, 339–55.

Porpora, D. (2007) Social structure. In Hartwig, M. (ed.) *Dictionary of Critical Realism*. London: Routledge, 422–5.

Porpora, D. (2015) *Reconstructing Sociology*. Cambridge: Cambridge University Press.

Porter, S. (2015a) Realist evaluation: an immanent critique, *Nursing Philosophy*, 16(4): 18–28.

Porter, S. (2015b) The uncritical realism of realist evaluation, *Evaluation*, 12(1): 65–82.

Porter, S. (2017) Evaluating realist evaluation: a response to Pawson's reply, *Nursing Philosophy*, 18(2): e12155.

Porter, S. and O'Halloran, P. (2012) The use and limitation of realistic evaluation as a tool for evidence-based practice: a critical realist perspective, *Nursing Inquiry*, 19(1): 18−28.

Porter, S., McConnell, T. and Reid, J. (2017a) The possibility of critical realist randomised controlled trials, *Trials*, 18(1).

Porter, S., McConnell, T., Clarke, M., Kirkwood, J., Hughes, N., Graham-Wisener, L., Regan, J., McKeown, M., McGrillen, K. and Reid, J. (2017b) A critical realist evaluation of a music therapy intervention in palliative care, *BMC Palliative Care*, 16(70), https://doi.org/10.1186/s12904-017-0253-5.

Posel, D. and Ross, F. C. (2014) Opening up the quandaries of research ethics: beyond the formalities of institutional ethical review. In Posel, D. and Ross, F. C. (eds) *Ethical Quandaries in Social Research*. Cape Town: HSRC Press, 1–26.

Price, L. (2016) Using retroduction to address wicked problems. In Næss, P. and Price, L. (eds) *Crisis System: A Critical Realist and Environmental Critique of Economics and the Economy*. London: Routledge, 109–29.

Profit, J., Lee, D., Zupancic, J. A., Papile, L., Gutierrez, C., Goldie, S., Gonzalez-Pier, E. and Salomon, J. (2010) Clinical benefits, costs, and cost-effectiveness of neonatal intensive care in Mexico, *PLoS Medicine*, 7(12): e1000379.

Pryor, J. (2010) Nurses create a rehabilitative milieu. *Rehabilitation Nursing*, 35(3): 123–8, http://search.ebscohost.com.ezproxy.aut.ac.nz/login.aspx?direct=true&db=cmedm&AN=20450021&site=ehost-live&scope=site.

Pryor, J. and Smith, C. (2002) A framework for the role of registered nurses in the specialty practice of rehabilitation nursing in Australia. *Journal of Advanced Nursing*, 39(3): 249–57, http://search.ebscohost.com/login.aspx?direct=true&db=rzh&AN=2002153668&site=ehost-live.

Purser, R. (2019) *McMindfulness: How Mindfulness Became the New Capitalist Spirituality*. London: Repeater.

Ravitsky, V. (2020) *Post-Covid Bioethics*. New York: Hastings Bioethics Forum.

RCP, Royal College of Physicians (2003) *Allergy: The Unmet Need. A Blueprint for Better Patient Care*. London: RCP.

RCP, Royal College of Physicians (2010) *Allergy Care: Still Not Meeting the Unmet Need*. London: RCP.

RCPCH, Royal College of Paediatrics and Child Health (2020) *State of Child Health*, https://www.rcpch.ac.uk/resources/state-of-child-health

RCPsych, Royal College of Psychiatrists (2014) *Report of the Second Round of the National Audit of Schizophrenia (NAS)*. London: RCPsych.

Rempel, E., Barnett, J. and Durrant, H. (2019) The hidden assumptions in public engagement: a case study of engaging on ethics in government data analysis, *Research for All*, 3(2): 180–90.

Retraction Watch (2019) http://retractiondatabase.org/RetractionSearch.aspx

Rhodes, L. (1991) *Emptying Beds: The Work of an Emergency Psychiatric Unit*. Berkeley, CA: University of California Press.

Riggs, K. and Greene, J. (2015) Why is there no generic insulin? *New England Journal of Medicine*, 372: 1171–5.

Rittel, H. and Webber, M. (1973) Dilemmas in a general theory of planning, *Policy Sciences*, 4(2): 155–69.

Røen, I., Stifoss-Hanssen, H., Grande, G., Brenne, A.-T., Kaasa, S., Sand, K. and Knudsen, A. (2018) Resilience for family carers of advanced cancer patients—how can health care providers contribute? A qualitative interview study with carers, *Palliative Medicine*, 32(8): 1410–18.

Rønnestad, M. et al (2018) Expanding the conceptualization of outcome and clinical effectiveness, *Journal of Contemporary Psychotherapy*, 49: 87–97, https://doi.org/10.1007/s10879-018-9405-z

Roosevelt, E. (1999 [1958]) Where do human rights begin? In Black, A. (ed.) *Courage in a Dangerous World*. New York: Columbia University Press.

Rose, H. and Rose, S. (2014) *Genes, Cells and Brains: The Promethean Promise of the New Biology*. London: Verso.

Rose, N. (1990) *Governing the Soul*. London: Free Association Books.

Roué, J.-M., Kuhn, P., Lopez Maestro, M., Maastrup, R., Mitanchez, D., Westrup, B. and Sizun, J. (2017) Eight principles for patient-centred and family-centred care for newborns in the neonatal intensive care unit, *Archives of Disease of Childhood: Fetal & Neonatal Edition*, 102(4): F364–8.

Ryan, F. (2019) *Crippled: Austerity and the Demonization of Disabled People*. London: Verso.

Sadler, M., Santos, M. And Ruiz-Berdún, D., Rojas, G., Skoko, E., Gillen, P. and Clausen, J. (2016) Moving beyond disrespect and abuse: addressing the structural dimensions of obstetric violence, *Reproductive Health Matters*, 24(47): 47–55.

Said, E. (1995) *Orientalism: Western Conceptions of the Orient*. London: Penguin.

Sainato, M. (2019) Medication or housing: why soaring insulin prices are killing Americans, *Guardian*, 23 September.

Saks, M. and Allsop, J. (eds) (2019) *Researching Health: Qualitative, Quantitative and Mixed Methods*. London: SAGE.

Sartre, J.-P. (1984) *Being and Nothingness: An Essay in Phenomenological Ontology*. New York: Washington Square Press.

Sayer, A. (1992) *Method in Social Science: A Realist Approach*. London: Routledge.

Sayer, A. (2000) *Realism and Social Science*. London: SAGE.

Sayer, A. (2009) Who's afraid of critical social science? *Current Sociology*, 57(6): 767–86.

Sayer, A. (2011) *Why Things Matter to People: Social Science, Values and Ethical Life*. Cambridge: Cambridge University Press.

Sayer, A. (2017) Normativity in the social sciences. In Kjorstad, M. and Solem, M. (eds) *Critical Realism for the Welfare Professions*. London: Routledge, 23–37.

Sayer, A. (2019) Normativity and naturalism as if nature mattered, *Journal of Critical Realism*, 18(258): 273.

Sayer, P. (2020) Policy and politics: a new understanding of evidence-based policy, *Discover Society*, 4 March.

Scambler, G. (2018) *Sociology, Health and the Fractured Society*. London: Routledge.

Schrecker, T. and Bambra, C. (2015) *How Politics Makes Us Sick: The Body Economic*. Basingstoke: Palgrave.

Schutt, R. (2006) *Investigating the Social World: The Process and Practice of Research*. Thousand Oaks, CA: SAGE.

Schutz, A. (1967) *The Phenomenology of the Social World*. Evanston, IL: Northwestern University Press.

Scott, S., Curnock, E., Mitchell, R., Robinson, M., Taulbut, M., Tod, E. and McCartney, G. (2013) *What Would It Take to Eradicate Health Inequalities? Testing the Fundamental Causes Theory of Health Inequalities in Scotland*. Glasgow: NHS Health Scotland.

Seabrook, J. (2015) *Pauperland: Poverty and the Poor in Britain*. London: Hurst.

Seidler, V. (1986) *Kant, Respect and Injustice*. London: Routledge.

Sen, A. (1999) *Development as Freedom*. Oxford: Oxford University Press.

Sentamu, J. (2019) Major global inquiry launches to address human and environmental impact of oil companies operating in Nigeria. York: Archbishop of York News.

Sewell, W. (1992) A theory of structure, *American Journal of Sociology*, 98(1): 1–29.

Shakespeare, T. (2010) The social model of disability. In Davis, L. (ed.) *The Disability Studies Reader*. New York: Routledge, 266–73.

Shakespeare, T. (2013) *Disability Rights and Wrongs Revisited*. London: Routledge.

Shakespeare, T., Watson, N. and Alghaib, A. (2017) Blaming the victim, all over again: Waddell and Aylward's biopsychosocial (BPS) model of disability, *Critical Social Policy*, 37(1): 22–41.

Sharfstein, S. (2005) Big pharma and American psychiatry: the good, the bad and the ugly, *American Psychiatric Association Psychiatric News*, https://doi.org/10.1176/pn.40.16.00400003

Shaxson, N. (2018) *The Finance Curse: How Global Finance Is Making Us All Poorer*. London: Vintage.

Shipton, E., Shipton, E. and Shipton, A. (2018) A review of the opioid epidemic: what do we do about it? *Pain and Therapy*, 7: 23–36.

Shove, E. and Spurling, N. (eds) (2013) *Sustainable Practices: Social Theory and Climate Change*. London: Routledge.

Shweder, R. (2006) Protecting human subjects and preserving academic freedom: prospects at the University of Chicago, *American Ethnologist*, 33: 507–18.

Silverman, D. (ed.) (1997) *Qualitative Research*. London: SAGE.

Silverman, D. (2009) *Interpreting Qualitative Data* (4th edn). London: SAGE.

Silverman, D. (2017) *Doing Qualitative Research*. London: SAGE,

Sironi, M., Ploubidis, G. and Grundy, E. (2020) Fertility history and biomarkers using prospective data: evidence from the 1958 National Child Development Study, *Demography*, 57: 529–58, https://doi.org/10.1007/s13524-020-00855-x

Skinningsrud, T. (2007) Realist social theorising and the emergence of state education system. In Lawson, C., Latsis, J. S. and Martin, N. (eds) *Contributions to Social Ontology*. London: Routledge, 252–72.

Smallwood, G. (2015) *Indigenist Critical Realism: Human Rights and First Australians' Wellbeing*. London: Routledge.

Smith, C. (2010) *What Is a Person? Rethinking Humanity, Social Life, and the Moral Good from the Person Up*. Chicago, IL: University of Chicago Press.

Smith, D. (2011) Pfizer pays out to Nigerian families of meningitis drug trial victims, *Guardian*, 12 August.

Smith, E. and Anderson, K. (2018) Understanding lay perspectives on socioeconomic health inequalities in Britain: a meta-ethnography, *Sociology of Health & Illness*, 409(1): 146–70.

Smith, K. and Stewart, E. (2017) We need to talk about impact: why social policy academics need to engage with the UK's research impact agenda, *Journal of Social Policy*, 46(1): 109–27.

Smith, K., Bambra, C. and Hill, S. (eds) (2016) *Health Inequalities: Critical Perspectives*. Oxford: Oxford University Press.

Smith, L. (2005) On tricky ground: researching the native in the age of uncertainty. In Denzin, N. and Lincoln, Y. (eds) *The SAGE Handbook of Qualitative Research*. Thousand Oaks, CA: SAGE, 85–108.

Snow, S. (2008) John Snow: the making of a hero? *Lancet*, 372: 22–3.

Spacey, A., Scammell, J., Board, M. and Porter, S. (2019) Systematic critical realist review of interventions designed to improve end-of-life care in care homes, *Nursing and Health Sciences*, 22(2): 343–54.

Stanley, L. and Wise, S. (2010) The ESRC's 2010 framework for research ethics: fit for research purpose? *Sociological Research Online*, 15(4): 106–15.

Suarez, E. and Gadalla, T. (2010) Stop blaming the victim: a meta-analysis of on rape myths, *Journal of Interpersonal Violence*, 25(11): 2010–35.

Sutcliffe, K., Melendez-Torres, G., Burchett, H., Richardson, M., Rees, R. and Thomas, J. (2018) The importance of service-users' perspectives: a systematic review of qualitative evidence reveals overlooked critical features of weight management programmes, *Health Expectations*, 21: 563–73.

Swenson, C. (2016) *DBT Principles in Action: Acceptance, Change and Dialectics*. New York: Guildford Press.

Taman, A. (2020) A dying shame, *The Lowdown*, 2 March, https://lowdownnhs.info/funding/a-dying-shame-marmot-throws-down-the-gauntlet-alan-taman/

Taylor, J. and Harvey, S. (2009) Effects of psychotherapy with people who have been sexually assaulted: a meta-analysis, *Aggression and Violent Behavior*, 14(5): 273–85.

Teeple, G. (2019) Foreword. In Bryant, T., Raphael, D. and Rioux, M. (eds) *Staying Alive: Critical Perspectives on Health, Illness, and Health Care*. Toronto: Canadian Scholars Press, vi–xiii.

Tew, J. (2011) *Social Approaches to Mental Distress*. Basingstoke: Palgrave MacMillan.

Therborn, G. (2014) *The Killing Fields of Inequality*. Cambridge: Polity.

Tilley, L. (2020) Saying the quiet part out loud: eugenics and the 'aging population' in Conservative pandemic governance, *Discover Society*, 6 April.

Toynbee, P. and Walker, D. (2020) *The Lost Decade 2010-2020 and What Lies Ahead for Britain*. London: Faber.

Turner, B. (2008) *The Body and Society*. London: SAGE.

Tseris, E. (2013) Trauma Theory Without Feminism? *Affilia*, 28(2): 153–64.

UN, United Nations (1948) *Universal Declaration of Human Rights*. New York: UN.

UN, United Nations (1966) *International Covenant on Economic, Social and Cultural Rights*. New York: UN.
UN, United Nations (1989) *Convention on the Rights of the Child*. Geneva: UNHCHR.
UNCTAD, United Nations Conference on Trade and Development (2019) Financing a global green new deal, https://unctad.org/en/pages/PublicationWebflyer.aspx?publicationid=2526
UNFAO, United Nations Food and Agriculture Organization (2019) *Annual State of Food and Agriculture Report*. New York: UNFAO.
Unger, R. (2007) *The Self Awakened: Pragmatism Unbound*. Cambridge, MA: Harvard University Press.
UNICEF (2005) The baby-friendly hospital initiative, https://www.unicef.org/nutrition/index_24806.html
Urry, J. (2011) *Climate Change & Society*. Cambridge: Polity.
Valentini, L. (2017) Dignity and human rights: a reconceptualisation, *Oxford Journal of Legal Studies*, 37(4): 862–85.
Vincent, S. and Wapshott, R. (2014) Critical realism and the organisational case study: A guide to discovering institutional mechanism. In Edwards, P., O'Mahoney, J. and Vincent, S. (eds) *Putting Critical Realism into Practice: A Guide to Research Methods in Organization Studies*. Oxford: Oxford University Press, 148–67.
Wadley, J. (2015) Online survey researchers should be cautious with trick questions, *Michigan University News*, 26 May.
Warner, J. and Spitters, S. (2017) Integrating care for children with allergic diseases: UK experience, *Current Allergy Clinical Immunology*, 30: 172–8.
Wasco, S. (2003) Conceptualizing the Harm done by Rape, *Trauma, Violence, & Abuse*, 4(4): 309–322.
Wassenaar, D. and Mamotte, N. (2012) Ethical issues and ethics reviews in social science research. In Leach, M., Stevens, M., Lindsay, G., Ferrero, A. and Korkut, Y. (eds) *The Oxford Handbook of International Psychological Ethics*. Oxford: Oxford University Press, 268–82.
Weber, M. (1968) *Economy and Society: An Outline of Interpretive Sociology*. New York: Bedminster Press.
Weinberg, C. (2020) Punishment is the pandemic, *Abolition Journal*, 11 May, https://abolitionjournal.org/punishment-is-the-pandemic/
Weizenegger, B. (2020) 'What do you do that's so special, anyway?': an examination of the mechanisms of change in feminist-informed sexual assault counselling. Doctoral dissertation in progress. Melbourne: University of Melbourne.

White, R. (2007) Institutional review board mission creep: the common rule, social science, and the nanny state, *The Independent Review*, 11: 547–64.

Whitehead, D. (2010) Health promotion in nursing: a Derridean discourse analysis, *Health Promotion International*, 26(1): 117–27.

WHO, World Health Organization (2011) *Tackling Antibiotic Resistance from a Food Safety Perspective in Europe*. Copenhagen: WHO.

WHO, World Health Organization (2019a) *Health Statistics and Information Systems: Global Health Estimates*. Geneva: WHO, https://www.who.int/healthinfo/global_burden_disease/en/

WHO, World Health Organization (2019b) Measles and rubella surveillance data, https://www.who.int/immunization/monitoring_surveillance/burden/vpd/surveillance_type/active/measles_monthlydata/en/

Wilkinson, R. and Pickett, K. (2009) *The Spirit Level: Why More Equal Societies Almost Always Do Better*. London: Allen Lane.

Wilkinson, R. and Pickett, K. (2015) Income inequality and health: a causal review, *Social Science & Medicine*, 128: 316–26.

Wilkinson, R. and Pickett, K. (2018) *The Inner Level*. London: Allen Lane.

Williams, M. (2008) Review essay: an orchestra of soloists, *Sociology*, 42: 1023–8.

Williams, O. (2020) Revealed: Palantir commits 45 engineers to NHS coronavirus data project, earns £1, https://tech.newstatesman.com/coronavirus/palantir-45-engineers-to-nhs-covid-19-datastore

Willow, C. (2019) When the state says it's all right to hurt a child, *Open Democracy*, 8 August, https://www.opendemocracy.net/en/shine-a-light/when-the-state-says-its-all-right-to-hurt-a-child/

Winch, P. (1958) *The Idea of a Social Science and Its Relations to Philosophy*. London: Routledge and Kegan Paul.

WOF, World Obesity Federation (2019) The first global atlas on childhood obesity, https://www.worldobesity.org/nlsegmentation/global-atlas-on-childhood-obesity

WOF, World Obesity Federation (2020) Obesity is a disease statement, https://www.worldobesity.org/about/about-obesity.

Wong, G., Greenhalgh, T., Westhorp, G., Buckingham, J. and Pawson, R. (2013) RAMESES publication standards: meta-narrative reviews, *Journal of Advanced Nursing*, 69: 987–1004.

Woodiwiss, A. (2005) *Human Rights*. London: Routledge.

Worell, J. and Remer, P. (2002) *Feminist Perspectives in Therapy: An Empowerment Model for Women*. New York: Wiley.

World Food Programme (2019) Hunger map, https://www.wfp.org/publications/2019-hunger-map

Wright, E. O. (2010) *Envisioning Real Utopias*. London: Verso.

Wright, T. (2012) *Circulation: William Harvey's Revolutionary Idea*. London: Chatto.

Wyatt, L. (2019) *A History of Nursing*. Stroud: Amberley.

Wylie, C. (2019) *Mindf*ck: Inside Cambridge Analytica's Plot to Break the World*. London: Profile.

Ye, Y., Chen, N., Chen, J., Liu, J., Lin, L., Liu, Y., Lang, Y., Li, X., Yang, X. and Jiang, X. (2015) Internet-based cognitive–behavioural therapy for insomnia (ICBT-i): a meta-analysis of randomised controlled trials, *BMJ Open*, 6: e010707.

Yin, R. (2014) *Case Study Research: Design and Methods*. London: SAGE.

Young, M. and Muller, J. (2016) *Curriculum and the Specialization of Knowledge*. London: Routledge.

Zhang, W., Robertson, J., Jones, A., Dieppe, P. and Doherty, M. (2008) The placebo effect and its determinants in osteoarthritis: meta-analysis of randomized controlled trials, *Annals of Rheumatic Disease*, 67: 1716–23.

Žižek, S. (2014) Fat-free chocolate and absolutely no smoking: why our guilt about consumption is all-consuming, *Guardian*, 21 May.

Index of subjects

Note: Page numbers for tables appear in italics.

1M 153–4, 155, 159, 160, 161, *162*, 163, 165
2E 153, 154–5, 159, 160, 161, *162*, 164, 165
3L 153, 155–7, 159, 160, 161, *162*, 164
4D 157–9, 160, 161, *162*, 164–5

A

absence 121, 146–8, 151, 154–5, 164, 173, 182
actor network theory (ANT) 75–7, 81, 117
actual 49, 50, 51, 53, 54, *60*, *85*, 182
agency 18, 32, 55, 66–7, 68–79, 81–92, 132
  and behaviourism 47
  and interdisciplinary work 142
  and naturalism 49
agents 32, 67, 68, 146
air pollution 14
allergies 163–5
anaesthesia 11, 12, 13
antibiotics 172
antisepsis 13
antithesis 48, 150, 152, 185
asthma 164–5
austerity 19, 37, 82, 97, 129, 177
  and premature deaths 19
  and prisons 157
autonomous reflexivity 90

B

babies 53–4, 107, 141–2, 160, 162–3
basic critical realism (BCR) 121
behaviourism 47, 96, *139*
behaviour-modifying programmes 16
benign MELD 159, 161
Bhopal 79
bioethics 113–14
bio-psycho-social models 132

C

cancer 13, 46
capitalism 135–6
care
  integrated 36–8, 164, 165
  intensive 53–5, 76, 78, 141, 160, 162
  status 142
  terminal 72
causality 18, 34, 155
causal mechanisms 49–50, 51–2, 54, 55, 57, *85*, 108
  and agents 81, 84
  definition 182
  and mental health services 178
  and Porter 83
central conflation 82
change, transformative 145–66, 186
chemotherapy 13, 172
children 32, 52, 53, 59, 75, 124, 163–5
  and consent 60
  in poverty 145
  rights 103
  and Sure Start 17, 18
  and vaccinations 67, 113–14
chloroform 11
cholera 11
class/command dynamic 121, 122
closed systems 15, 44–5, 46, 48, 182
CMO (context-mechanism-outcome) 27, 29, 31, 32–3, 82, 83
Cochrane Collaboration 19

cognitive behaviour therapy 68–9
collectivism 61
communicative reflexivity 90
community-based integrated care service 36–8
community mental health team (CMHT) 177
concrete 136, 137, 146, 156, 182
concrete<–>universal singular 90, 137, 156, 182
conflation 81–2
consent 59–60, 71–2, 108–9, 113
constant conjunctions 16, 45, 52, 80
constellations 156, 183
constructionists 22, 27, 42, 97, 107–8
contexts 30, 31, 32, 33, 36, 70, 71
  and 3L 153
  and agents 146
  and ANT 76
  definition 29
  and interpretivists 98
  local 108
  and TMSA 84–5
  and totality 174
  and values 97
contradictions 58, 93, 137, *139*, 159, 160, 162
  and absence 155
  definition 183
  and emergence 149
  and immanent critique 77, 150
conversation analysis (CA) 74–5
conversations, inner 90
cortisol 57
counselling 134
covering law 16, 17, 80, 183
covert power 56
COVID-19 pandemic 1, 2, 19, 136–7, 168, 169, 172
  and interdisciplinary work 170–1
  and reductionists 47
critical discourse analysis 75
critical philosophy 77–8
critical social science (CSS) 109–10
cross-infection, prevention 2, 3
cultural relativism 97–8
culture 78–9, 183

D

deception 108
deduction 11, 42, 55, *139*
Delhi 14
demi-regs 45, 46, 183
Democratic Republic of Congo (DRC) 167
deontology 43, 114, *115*
determinism 81–2, 91
diabetes 13, 50, *51*, 52, 89
dialectic 83–8, 146, 150, 160, 183
dialectical critical realism (DCR) 121, 150–9, 183
Dialectic and Difference 148
Dialectic: The Pulse of Freedom 160
difference 148–9
dignity 105–7
directional interaction 87
disability 110–11
disabled people 68, 110, 116, 139–40
disadvantage 156, 158
discourse 36–7, 38, 75, 150
disembodiment 71
distorted communication 122
distress 133–5
downward conflation 81–2
drugs 101, 136, 167

E

Ebola epidemics 98
eclecticism *139*
Economic Rescue Plan for All 172
education policy 168–9
emergence 149, 183
empirical 49, 50, 51, 53, *60*, *85*, 183
empiricism *139*
endism 159, 183

Engager 86–8
Enlightened Common Sense 151
epistemic fallacy *139*, 150, 151, 183
epistemological relativism 175
epistemology 42–3, 183
equality 12, 34, 63, 102, 111, 124, *139*
ethical naturalism 118–19, 183
ethics 112–19, 124
ethnographers 97
ethnography 72, 97
ethnomethodology 59–60, 74, 81
eudaimonic society 114, 175, 183
eugenics 12, 19
evolution 49–50
explicit power 56

F
Factory Act, 1867 58
facts 98–9, *139*, 172, 175
Family-Nurse Partnership (FNP) 124
feminist counselling 134
fetish 160–1, 183
field 68
flat actualism 52, 75, 182
four planes of social being 128–32, 136–7, 142–3, 183
fractured reflexivity 90
freedom 109–10
functionalism 31, 63, 97, *139*, 183
futures 173

G
generative mechanisms 50, 57, 58–60, 70, 183
Glasgow 158
global heating 14
gold standard *139*
greenhouse gases 14
grounded theory 72–3

H
habitus 68, 80, 81
half-regularities 45
happiness 69, 70, 71
The Health of the Nation 96
health visitors 124
heart surgery 59, 60
hegemony 69, 183
herd immunity 2
hermeneutics 47–8, 61, 183
hermeticism 78, 183
hierarchy *139*
homo economicus 68
human rights 102–5, 106, 111

I
I, Daniel Blake 82
idealism 42, 47, 186
identity 90, 152
 see also non-identity
immanent, definition 183
immanent critique 77, 149–50, 160, 183
impersonal power 56
India 14, 79
individualism 61
induction 11, *139*
institutional review boards (IRBs) 113
insulin 13
integrated care 36–8, 164, 165
interactionism, symbolic 71
interdisciplinarity 136–40
interdisciplinary research and policymaking 135–6, 142, 170–1
internalised power 56
interpretivism 22–5, 26, 42, 49, 52, 59, 61, 62–3
 and agency within structures 71–3
 definition 184
 and ethics *118*
 and naturalism 47
interpretivism-hermeneutics 47–8
interpretivists 44, 48, 98
intransitive 43–4, 184
irrealism *139*, 184

J

judgemental rationality 142

K

knife crime 158

L

laminated 130, 184
laminated systems analysis 132–5
lifeworld 121–2, 123
London 14

M

malign MELD 159–61
materialism 150, 151, 184
MBA (Mentalisation-Based Approach) 86, 87
measles 45
mechanisms 32, 33, 36–7, 48, 83, 134, 163
  definition 29–30
  and demi-regs 45
  see also causal mechanisms
medical power 56
medicine 13, 15, 55
MELD 153–66, 176, 184
mental distress 177–8
mental health 86, 128–9, 176–8
mental illness 130–2
meta-reflexivity 90
metatheories 111–12, 172
Mexico 53–5, 160, 162–3
milk 160–1
mindfulness 68–9, 70
mini-MELDs 161–5
monovalence 148, 184
morality 98, 118
moral realism 119, 184
moral relativism 97
morphogenesis 85–8, 91–2, 142, 146, 155, 184
morphostasis 85–8, 184
mothers 53, 54, 56, 103, 160, 162–3
multidisciplinarity 137–8

N

naturalism 46–9, 118–19, 137, *139*, 176, 184
natural necessity 49–55, 60, 85, 108, 148, 184
negation 154–5, 184
neoliberalism 69, 70, 120
neonatal intensive care units (NICUs) 43, 53–5, 141, 160–1, 162–3
neonatal research 118–19
neurons 134
New Zealand 91
NHS staff, assaults against 106
non-identity 153–4, 163, 184
Nuremberg Code 103
nurses 78, 91–2, 160–1

O

obesity 13, 136
objectivity 42, 96, 172
offenders 31, 86
ontological realism 175
ontology 42–3, 44, 66, 81, 89, 133, 150
  definition 184
  and human rights 104
open systems 16, 33, 34, 45, 46, 48, 146
  and agency 49
  definition 184
outcomes 27, 29, 30, 31, 52, 136
  and MELD 159
  and utilitarians 97, 114

P

paradigms 12, 23, 24, 38, 40, 184
parenthood 19
parents 67, 74, 112, 124, 148, 159
  and consent 59, 60
  and neonatal intensive care units 43, 53, 54, 141, 160, 161, 162–3
penicillin 13
pensions, state 58

The Philosophical Foundation of the Three Sociologies 62
philosophy, critical 77–8
placebo 16
Planet of Slums 176
policy, health researchers' difficulties with 62
political economy 57–8
polyvalence 146–7, 148, 157, 184
positivism 42, 47–8, 49, 52, 61
  and agency within structures 68–71
  definition 184
  and ethics *118*
  and policy 62
positivists 15–17, 44, 63, 98–9, 101
poverty 14, 95, 145, 156, 158
power 56, 68, 107, 117, 121, 134, 160
  and agency 84
  and causal mechanisms 108
  and discourse 37
  and functionalists 97
power1 56, 84, 105, 146, 184
power2 69, 84, 105, 110, 146, 154, 157
  definition 56, 184
praxis 89, 152, 157, 160, 164–5, 184
presence 146–8, 151
prisoners 31
prison leavers 86–8, 157
prisons 1, 157
psychiatric units 128–9

R

radical negation 154
randomisation 15, 16
rationality 142
RCTs (randomised controlled trials) 15, 16, 19, 20–1, 29, 45, 46
  and consent 113–14
  and FNP 124
realism 26–34, 48, *139*, 175, 185, 186
realist evaluation (RE) 26–34, 36–8, 82–3
reality-ontology 81
REC-IRB review 115–16
reductionism 46–7, *139*, 185
referent 44, 148, 150
reflexivity 90, *139*
regressions 16
rehabilitation 91–2
reification 160, 185
relativism 97–8, *139*, 175
research ethics committees (RECs) 113
retroduction 11–12, 55, 185
rights 102–5, 106, *109*, 111

S

Scientific Advisory Group for Emergencies (SAGE) 47
scientism *139*, 185
Scotland 158
Seguro Popular 54
semi-closed systems 33
semiotics 44
semiotic triangle 44, 151, 185
SEPM (synchronic emergent powers materialism) 89, 185
serious mental illness (SMI) 130–2
sexual assault 132–5
shareholders 127–8
signifiers 44
signs 44
social causal mechanisms 83
  see also causal mechanisms
social construction 110, 141
social constructionists 97, 107–8
social constructivism 73–4
social structure, agency and culture (SAC) 81
social structures 27, 79–81, 82, 83, 140, 156, 178
  and Charlie Gard 112
  and interpretivism 47
  presented as 'variables' 18
space 147, 155, 156, 159, 182
stasis 85, 151
state pensions 58
strategic action 122
stress 37, 57, 65, 70, 172
structural determinism 81–2

structures 66–7, 68–93, 142, 178, 185
suicide 47
Sure Start 17, 18
surveillance 56, 69
symbolic interactionism 71
synchronic 89, 185
synthesis 150, 155, 156–7, 185
synthesised reviews 20–1
systematically distorted communication 122
systematic reviews 20, 21

T

tacit beliefs 18–19, 62
tacit theories *139*
telos 107
temporal interactions 87
tendencies 27, 45, 46, 48, 92, 173, 176
  definition 185
  and demi-regs 183
  and transfactual 186
tensed 146, 155, 156, 185
textual discourse analysis 150
theory-practice consistency 84, 185
thesis 150, 152, 153, 185
thrownness 84, 185
time, and change 145–65
TINA (There Is No Alternative) 120, 149–50, 159, 185
TMSA (transformational model of social activity) 84–5, 142, 146, 154, 155, 186
totality 155–7, 164, 165, 174, 186
Trans-Atlantic US-UK trade deal 135–6
transcendental idealism 47, 186
transcendental realism 48, 175, 186
transfactual 48, 51–2, 137, 142, 156, 186
transformative change 145–66, 186
transformative negation 154
transitive 43, 44, 186
trust 86, 87, 108–9, 172–3
truth 107–9, 172

U

UK
  and health inequalities 57
  and Trans-Atlantic trade deal 135–6
UN Convention on the Rights of the Child (UNCRC) 103
under-labouring 77
Union Carbide tragedy 79
Universal Declaration of Human Rights (UDHR) 103, 105
upward conflation 82
US
  and health inequalities 57
  and Trans-Atlantic trade deal 135–6
utilitarianism 114, *115*
utilitarians 97
utility 114
utopia 174–5, 176

V

vaccines 13, 67, 113–14
value-freedom 96–8
values 98–102, 109–13, 123, 124–5, *139*
veils 160
Verstehen 22, 97
virtue ethics 114–15
voluntarism 82, 91

W

water 14, 109
wealth 14
webs of illusion 160
weight-reducing courses 16
wicked problems 39, 50, 186
World Obesity Forum 136

Y

young people 52, 98, 128–9, 155, 158

Index of names

Note: Page numbers for tables appear in italics.

A

Adam, B. 173
Ancel, P.-Y. 53
Archer, M. 8, 78, 80, 81, 85, 88, 89, 177
  and inner conversations 90
  on preverbal learning 107
Arendt, H. 158
Aristotle 150
Arnaud, C. 53

B

Bambra, C. 57, 119, 179
Bartley, M. 119
Bauman, Z. 158
Bentham, J. 69, 114
Benton, T. 62
Bhaskar, R. 7, 33, 47–8, 61, 82, 121, 158
  on agency 89
  on causal mechanisms 51–2
  on dialectic 153, 160
  on disability 111–12
  on disabled people 139–40
  on eudaimonia 114
  on immanent critique 149
  on Nietzsche 99
  on open systems 45
  on philosophers 147
  on semiotic triangle 44
  and TMSA 84–5
  on totality 155, 157
  on utopia 175
Blalock, H. 17
Blaxter, M. 23
Bourdieu, P. 68, 69, 120
British Medical Journal 24
Buckingham, J. 29, 30, 34
Bury, M. 23
Byng, R. 86–8

C

Case, A. 135
Claris, O. 53
Clegg, S. 21
Common Wealth 171
Comte, A. 31
Coquelin, A. 53
Cornwall, A. 22
Cunningham, B. 28, 30, 31
Cuttini, M. 53

D

Dalkin, S. 28, 30, 31
Danermark, B. 111–12, 139–40
Davenport, A. 91–2
Davies, W. 69, 70
Davis, M. 176
Deaton, A. 135
Deleuze, G. 71
Denzin, N. 117
Derrida, J. 150
De Tocqueville, A. 170
De Vries, J. 117
Dickson, K. 33, 34, 35
Dorling, D. 95
Doshi, P. 113–14
D'Souza, R. 174–5
Durkheim, E. 31, 47, *63–4*, 68, 79
Durox, M. 53

E

Edwards, P 20–1
Engels, F. 150–1

F

Fisher, M. 70
Fonagy, P. 88–9
Foucault, M. 56, 69
Fox, D. 119, 179
Fox, N. 22
Fox, R. 117–18
Frank, A. 23–4

G

Gard, C. 112
Garfinkel, H. 74
Garrett, L. 167
Gaventa, J. 22
Gearty, C. 111
Geertz, C. 71
Giardina, M. 117
Giddens, A. 82
Girma, H. 110
Glaser, B. 72–3
Glorieux, I. 53
Goffman, E. 71, 72
Goodfield, J. 101
Gough, D. 20, 124
Greenhalgh, J. 28
Greenhalgh, T 29, 30, 31, 34
Green Hofer, S. 130–1
Guattari, F. 71
Guba, Y. 24–5
Guterres, A. 170–1

H

Habermas, J. 121–2, 123
Hammersley, M. 100
Hartnell, N. 78
Harvey, D. 55, 120, 174
Harvey, W. 41
Hegel, G.W.F. 150
Henley, L. 117
Heraclitus 148
Hérbert, P. 115
Hinds, K. 33, 34, 35
Horton, R. 2
Huang, C. et al 2
Hume, D. 16, 45, 47, 61, 98–9

I

Ioannidis, J. 20

J

Jagosh, J. 31
Johnson, P. 136
Jones, D 28, 30, 31

K

Kaminski, M. 53
Kant, I. 47
Keller, E. 101
Kendrick, H. 36–8, 75
Khoshnood, B. 53
Klein, N. 120
Krieger, N. 58
Kuhn, T. 40

L

Latour, B. 76
Law, J. 75
Lawson, T. 45
Layard, R. 69
Lee, E. 75
Levitas, R. 174
Lhussier, M. 28, 30, 31
Lincoln, E. 24–5
Locke, J. 6
Lowe, P. 75
Lukes, S. 56

M

Macklin, R. 106
Mamotte, N. 117
Manzano, A. 31
Marmot, M. 101–2
Marteau, T. 97
Martin, K. 128–9
Marx, K. *63–4*, 150–1, 168
Mavarish, J. 75
McCarraher, E. 68
McCoy, D. 169
McDonnell, O. 22
McKie, R. 167
Mead, M. 97–8
Mendizabal-Espinosa, R. 53–5, 118–19

Midgley, M. 6
Mill, J. 114
Mire, S. 98
Mirowski, P. 120
Molyneux, J. 151
Morgan, J. 89
Moth, R. 176–8

N

Næss, P. 46
NAO (National Audit Office) 95
Norrie, A. 148
Nussbaum, M. 110

O

O'Hara, M. 95
Oliver, S. 20, 124
O'Mahony, J. 20–1
Oxfam 172

P

Paine, T. 104
Parker, J. 142
Parmenides 147
Parsons, T. 31, 68
Pauli, B. 109
Pawson, R. 28, 30, 31, 32, 33, 34, 39
  on mechanisms 29
  and Porter 82–3
  on values 123
Pickett, K. 56–7
Pierrat, V 53
Pilgrim, D. 74
Place, B. 76
Plato 148
Porpora, D. 6, 79, 80, 142, 172–3
Porter, S. 82–3, 123–4, 161–2
Price, L. 39

R

Roosevelt, E. 104
Rose, N. 69
Rosen, W. 115
Ryan, A. 114
Rybczynska-Bunt, S. 86–8

S

Sayer, A. 8, 99–100, 109–10, 119
Scambler, G. 120–3
Scott-Samuel, A. 119, 179
Shakespeare, T. 110
Snow, Dr J. 11, 12
Spitters, S. 163–5
Strauss, A. 72–3

T

Teeple, G. 65, 66
Thatcher, M. 80
Thomas, J. 20, 124
Tilley, N. 28, 30, 32
Turner, B. 73–4

U

UN (United Nations) 107
UNCTAD (UN Conference on Trade and Development) 171
Unger, R. 173
Urry, J. 169–70, 173

V

Valentini, L. 106
Victoria, Queen 11, 12
Vincent, S. 20–1
Virchos, R. 169

W

Wassenaar, D. 117
Weber, M. *63–4*, 82
Weizenegger, B. 132–5
Westhorp, G. 29, 30, 31, 34
Weston, L. 86–8
WHO (World Health Organization) 2, 167, 171
Wilkinson, R. 56–7
Williams, M. 38
Wong, G. 29, 30, 31, 34
Wright, O. 173

Z

Žižek, S. 69